THE BIG 15 KETOGENIC DIET COOKBOOK

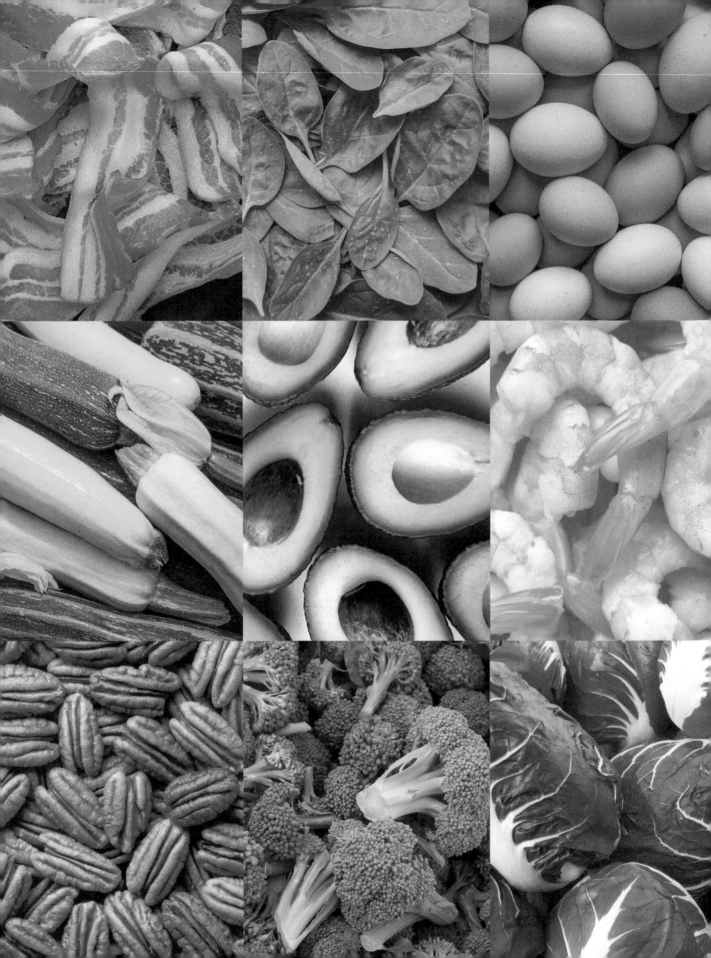

THE
BIG 15
KETOGENIC
DIET
COOKBOOK

15 Fundamental Ingredients
150 Keto Diet Recipes
300 Low-Carb & High-Fat Variations

MEGAN FLYNN PETERSON

ROCKRIDGE
PRESS

For general information on our other products and services or to obtain technical support, please contact our Customer Care Department within the United States at (866) 744-2665, or outside the United States at (510) 253-0500.

Rockridge Press publishes its books in a variety of electronic and print formats. Some content that appears in print may not be available in electronic books, and vice versa.

TRADEMARKS: Rockridge Press and the Rockridge Press logo are trademarks or registered trademarks of Callisto Media Inc. and/or its affiliates, in the United States and other countries, and may not be used without written permission. All other trademarks are the property of their respective owners. Rockridge Press is not associated with any product or vendor mentioned in this book.

All photography © Linda Schneider except SosnaRadosna/Shutterstock.com, cover, pp.ii & 22; Ataly/Shutterstock.com, cover, pp.ii, vi (spinach) & 194; Melanie Defazio/Stocksy, cover, pp.ii & 8; Aksana Yasiuchenia/Shutterstock.com, cover, pp.ii & 208; Toma Evsiukova/Stocksy, cover, pp.ii & 34, back cover; Jiri Hera/Shutterstock.com, cover, pp.ii & 136; Matin/Shutterstock.com, cover, pp.ii, vi (nuts) & 62; S_Derevianko/Shutterstock.com, cover, pp.ii & 180; Francesco de Marco/Shutterstock.com, cover, pp.ii & 150; MmeEmil/iStock, p.xii; Dene398/iStock, cover, p.48 & back cover; Magrig/Shutterstock.com, cover & p.76; Katerina Maksymenko/Shutterstock.com, cover & p.92; Davide Illini/Stocksy, cover & p.106; Pixel Stories/Stocksy, cover, p.120 & back cover; Trent Lanz/Stocksy, cover & p.164; IGphotography/iStock, p.230.

ISBN: Print 978-1-939754-42-4
eBook 978-1-939754-43-1

TO MY AMAZING READERS,
WHO MAKE PROJECTS LIKE THIS ONE POSSIBLE

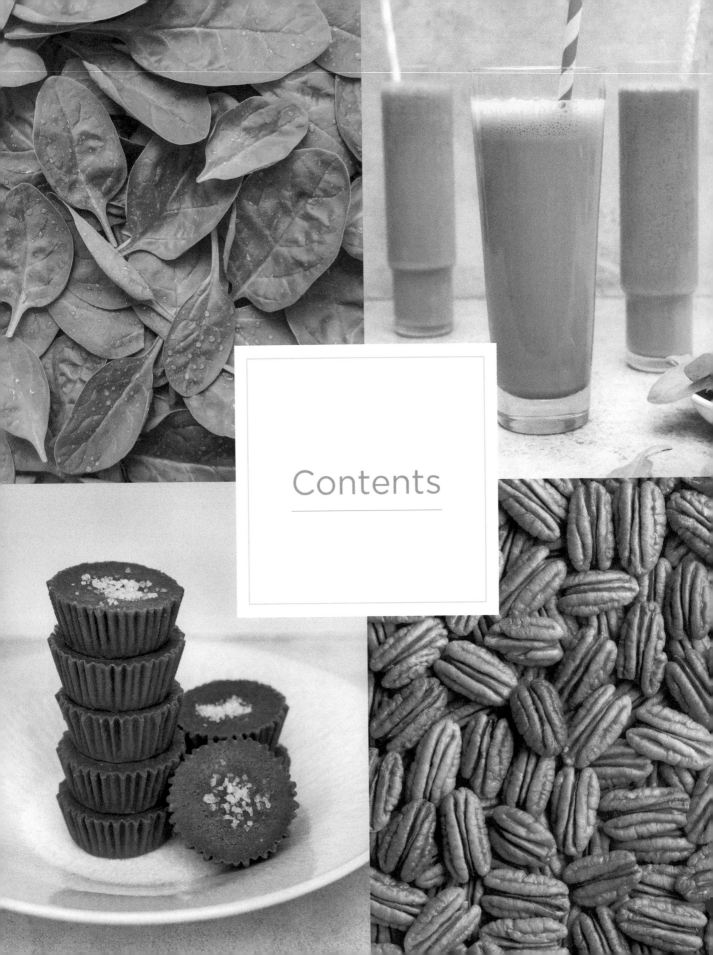

Contents

Introduction

If you've read my first two cookbooks, you know that I've followed a Paleo diet since November 2012. Learning about the Paleo diet was life-changing for me; my health and happiness really took an upward turn after learning (or un-learning) which foods were good for me and which ones made me feel worse.

I still really identify with the Paleo diet, and a lot of the tenets of a primal way of eating make so much sense to me, but after four or five years I was starting to gain weight again. Paleo is so easy to customize I found I was occasionally sneaking in sugar and rice, which then became gluten-free pasta or sandwich bread, and then I moved completely away from that to weekly beers with friends and other nonPaleo indulgences.

These slips started to become routines, and I realized that the whole "80/20" lifestyle didn't work for me. (That is, eating Paleo 80 percent of the time and "cheating" or treating myself to non-Paleo food 20 percent of the time.) Before I knew it, I had strayed completely from the Paleo diet and was eating way too much junk. I had fallen off the wagon without even realizing it, and I was struggling to get back on it.

Around this same time, one of my brothers-in-law began following a ketogenic diet, and my husband and I were blown away by his results. What was even more amazing to me than his weight loss was the fact that he managed to stick to the diet through the holidays. As a New Year's resolution, my husband and I decided to give it a try, and before I knew it I was losing weight, feeling better, and thinking about food and nutrition in a completely new way.

Paleo and keto diets have many similarities, but what I like (and needed) about keto is how precise and scientific it can be. At first glance, it seems incredibly restrictive and possibly even unrealistic. But if you think about it (and especially if you come from a Paleo background), the diet has a lot of mix-and-match qualities that I really appreciate.

You are allotted a certain number of carbs each day, and while that amount is very small, you can still pick and choose where they come from. Maybe it's a piece of fruit or a small scoop of ice cream. Either way, you can pick the foods you eat as long as they fit into your macros (macronutrients)—the things that make up the caloric content of a food. You may know them as fat, protein, and carbs, and to maintain a ketogenic diet your daily food consumption needs to consist of mostly fat, some protein, and very few carbs.

Generally, your daily rates will be in the following ranges:

- 60% to 75% of calories from fat
- 15% to 30% of calories from protein
- 5% to 10% of calories from carbs

Using a food calculator like MyFitnessPal to log your food for a few days will really help you plan your meals and snacks so you can hit your ideal ranges. If you look up a keto calculator online (see Resources, page 231), you can enter your height and weight and a few other pieces of information to get custom percentages based on your keto goals.

The hardest part about keto is definitely the beginning stage while you become keto adapted and finally enter ketosis. This doesn't usually take very long (just a few days), but drastically cutting carbs puts you in a state of sugar withdrawal (sometimes referred to as "carb flu"), which can be a little rough. You might have cravings for carbs or feel sluggish and/or irritable, but it will pass—just make sure to drink plenty of water and do your best to stick to the low-carb diet! If you cheat you'll draw out the process and make it a lot harder than if you just power through.

Keto works for me, and so I've written this book to help you embrace keto, too. The book is structured around familiar main ingredients, to make shopping and cooking a lot easier. The main ingredients range from big fats such as avocado, bacon, and dairy to proteins such as chicken and beef, to vegetables like spinach, broccoli, and cabbage. Most of the recipes are either main courses or side dishes, but there are some snacks and desserts thrown in as well. I've made sure to include good pairings here and there so you can match entrées with sides and create full meals; the mix-and-match nature of this book is intended to help you easily plan meals. The ingredient-based chapters are great for when you have something in your refrigerator and no idea what to do with it. And every recipe has two variations so you can get creative with flavors, textures, and cooking styles.

Now that I'm familiar with the two diets and their merits, I have found myself in "maintenance mode," going back and forth between them, creating what I refer to as a "low-carb, high-fat Paleo diet." But when it comes to weight loss, slimming down, and really getting your diet under control, keto is definitely the way to go.

LOW CARB, HIGH FAT, ALL NATURAL

The ketogenic (keto) diet is a low-carb, high-fat diet that makes losing weight really simple. It's important to balance the low-carbs with a high fat intake, which can seem a little counterintuitive if, like so many of us, you've grown up being told that fat makes you fat. But it's high-quality fats such as coconut oil, avocado, and butter from grass-fed cows that fuel your body once you enter ketosis—so fat is an incredibly important piece of the keto puzzle.

Ketosis is what makes keto work, so you should know that it's essentially the metabolic process in which the body stops using glucose (sugar) for energy and burns fats instead. Getting into ketosis involves more than just estimating and trying to eat as low-carb as possible, so do use a keto calculator online and enter your height, weight, estimated body fat percentage, and weight-loss goals. A calculator will give you a daily calorie count and your carb, fat, and protein macros. If you follow the guidelines, you'll reach and stay in a state of ketosis.

At first glance, the keto diet could appear to be full of "junk." After all, you eat a lot of cheese, butter, and oils. I'll admit this was the hardest thing for me to get used to, especially after years on the Paleo diet where I stayed away from dairy completely. But what you'll find in keto is that quality matters. You want high-fat, high-quality dairy and oils, preferably *grass-fed* and *organic* (if your budget allows). The diet is still mostly grain-free and absolutely free of added sugars—just like the Paleo diet.

After a few days on keto, I not only got used to the new rules but also ended up feeling glad that so much fat (especially dairy) was not just allowed but encouraged. Do keep in mind, though, that the ketogenic diet is certainly an alternative one, so make sure to talk to your health care provider about it if you have questions, especially if you have any health issues such as heart disease or high cholesterol.

THE EASIEST LOW-CARB DIET THERE IS

When I first started reading about keto, my initial thought was, *There's no way I'm going to be able to do this*, and I suspect it's the same for a lot of people. I used a keto calculator to figure out all my macros and, with my height and weight goal, I was allowed about 25 grams of carbs per day—that's the same amount of carbs as in one apple! But once you begin and get over that initial hump (a little sugar withdrawal combined with the thought, *What am I supposed to eat next?*), you'll find keto is actually very easy to stick to. This is what a typical day might look like for me in terms of meals and snacks:

- **Breakfast:** 2 bacon slices, Perfect Scrambled Eggs (page 10), ½ avocado
- **Snack:** Coconut Butter Coffee (page 224) or a cup of tea with coconut oil
- **Lunch:** Cobb Salad (page 81)
- **Snack:** Cheese Crisps (page 57), pork rinds, or raw veggies with Ranch Dressing (page 225).
- **Dinner:** Grilled steak or a cheeseburger without a bun—The Classic Juicy Lucy (page 102) would be perfect—plus a side salad with Ranch Dressing (page 225), and sautéed zucchini.
- **Dessert/Snack:** Small handful of raspberries or a Basic Sweet Fat Bomb (page 228).

BUT WAIT . . . IT'S NOT *THAT* EASY

While I'm a big advocate of the ketogenic diet being straightforward and accessible, it is true that there's a learning curve, and you really have to plan and be willing to cook. I would say that planning and cooking are most certainly among the hardest parts—there are very few keto-friendly takeout options!

Luckily for you, you're reading this book, so you already know what to make and eat! Planning your meals ahead and always having snacks on hand will make your life on the ketogenic diet a lot easier and is definitely the key to keto success. You'll also want to track everything you eat through an app such as MyFitnessPal or something similar; that way you can see what your day looks like and begin to learn which foods work for your goals.

REAL FOOD, REALLY SIMPLE

Because keto has become such a popular diet, there are a number of differing opinions on what is and isn't keto, how to balance macros, and best practices for generally implementing the diet into one's lifestyle in a way that's both effective and sustainable. It can take a lot of prep work to eat this way, and when so many recipes out there have numerous ingredients and long cooking times, it might seem almost impossible to come up with meals that work for you.

As noted already, there's a learning curve when it comes to keto, but other than that, the diet isn't a mystery—it's just smart eating using basic, familiar ingredients. The sooner you identify the most nutritious, keto-valuable food groups, the easier it will be for you to start eating well on the diet. Once you know what's what and get used to it all, living on the diet will come easily to you.

Take me, for example—I know that to stay in ketosis I need to eat about 25 grams of carbs (7% of the day's allotment), 76 grams of protein (21%), and 114 grams of fat (72%) every day. After a few weeks, I learned what I needed to get from the grocery store to meal plan one week at a time so I could hit those numbers every day. I learned which breakfasts worked, what I should have for lunch, good ideas for dinner, and what kinds of snack I should have between meals (if any—keto food is super filling and you'll probably find yourself eating less frequently than you used to).

This book will help you in two key ways:

1. It's full of keto-friendly recipes that offer meal ideas and help you plan your diet in a way that's organized and effective, so you know what to buy at the grocery store and how to cook it so it's delicious and nutritious.

2. Nutritional info is included with the recipes and variations to make calculating your macros that much easier. (When I first started, I had to log every single ingredient into MyFitnessPal to make sure my macros added up the way they were supposed to.) If you stick to the meals and snacks in this book it should be very easy to track everything and be that much closer to reaching your goals.

TIME-SENSITIVE, BUDGET-FRIENDLY

I've said it before and I'll say it again: If you're going to eat a special diet, you're going to have to cook. This is especially true for keto (and Paleo) diets. Because you'll be spending more time grocery shopping and cooking than you might be used to, most recipes in this book can be made in 30 minutes or fewer. If something takes longer than 30 minutes, it's probably a larger recipe or one that will last you longer than a few meals, which will save you time later in the week. You're busy; you want to spend time with your family and friends or doing the things that interest you, and spending hours in the kitchen may not be something that sounds fun.

You won't find any hard-to-come-by ingredients either, and I've kept to a minimum any recipes that include almond flour or specialty ingredients that can raise your grocery bill. I like cooking with straightforward, everyday ingredients that fit my values. I hope you'll find this helpful as you start your keto journey.

EAT THIS, LESS OF THAT, AND NONE OF THOSE

Keto is great because it's pretty customizable—if you don't tolerate dairy or want to stay Paleo you can just avoid cheese, heavy cream, and other dairy products, but otherwise you could look at the diet, basically, as a low-carb, high-fat version of the Paleo diet. It's grain-free, sugar-free, and, with the exception of dairy, generally free of most processed and/or packaged foods. Here's a list to get you started.

ENJOY

- Avocado
- Bone broth
- Butter and ghee
- Coconut oil
- Condiments: mayonnaise, mustard, pesto, pickles, and fermented foods such as kimchi and sauerkraut
- Dairy products, full-fat, such as cheese and heavy cream
- Eggs
- Fatty fish and seafood
- Grass-fed beef
- Leafy greens, including spinach and kale
- Most nonstarchy vegetables, including zucchini, summer squash, cucumber, and celery
- Pasture-raised lamb, pork, and poultry
- Some nuts: almonds, macadamias, pecans
- Water, black coffee, and tea

LIMIT

Limiting these foods will look different for every individual based on the rest of their diet—for example, someone who sweetens their morning coffee with Stevia every day is going to have less carbs left to also indulge in the occasional glass of dry wine or piece of dark chocolate. A lot of this also depends on whether you're actively trying to lose weight or have reached a maintenance stage of keto, where you can allow a few more carbs than you usually would. To make sure your macros are right (and to help you figure out what you have room for in your diet), stick to consistent tracking of your food intake and make sure your weight and goals are always updated in an app like MyFitnessPal or your favorite food/weight tracker.

WATER MAKES IT WORK

Drinking enough water is probably one of the most important things to remember when transitioning to keto (and once you're keto-adapted). Hydrate all day. Cutting down on carbs removes extra stores of water in your body, so it's easy to get dehydrated if you don't stay on top of your water consumption. Pay attention to symptoms such as increased thirst, dry mouth, headache, dizziness, or lethargy.

I like to sip water from a big beer glass throughout the day, regularly refilling it.

Other people have a special water bottle that keeps them on top of their intake. If you're not a plain water fan, add lemon, cucumber, mint, lime, or some combination to make it more interesting. I also love sparkling water—just make sure it's a brand that doesn't add any sugar or juice, such as LaCroix.

Not only is getting enough water important for hydration, it also helps curb cravings, keeps you from overeating, and is just generally great for your overall health.

- Alcohol, to dry red and white wines or liquors (without sugary mixers)
- Bacon and sausage with lots of preservatives and added sugars
- Berries
- Cocoa and dark chocolate
- Edamame

- Gluten-free soy sauce (or tamari)
- Low-carb sweeteners, such as stevia
- Most nuts
- Nightshades (eggplant, peppers, tomatoes)
- Starchy root vegetables, such as pumpkin or sweet potato

AVOID

- Anything that says "low fat" or "nonfat"
- Alcohol: Beer, sugary cocktails, sweet wines
- Grains of all types

- Milk, especially skim
- Most fruit and fruit juices
- Processed foods, such as almond milk and dried fruit
- Sweeteners

GO-TO PANTRY ITEMS

I've found a lot of variety in keto recipes, which is nice, but you still need a well-stocked pantry so you don't get bored after a few weeks of eating lots of the same things (when you find meals and macros that work well, it can be easy to get stuck in a rut rather than experiment all over again).

Following are the fats, herbs, oils, nuts, and spices you'll always find in my pantry and/or refrigerator; consider adding them to yours.

- Garlic (either whole, minced, or in powder form)
- Grass-fed butter
- Nut butters, such as almond or peanut
- Oils: Coconut, olive, and sesame
- Onion (either whole, dried, or in powder form)
- Sesame seeds
- Tomato paste (useful for making quick sauces or adding to casseroles)

ON MEATS, SWEETS, AND BUTTER

Throughout the recipes, you'll see certain ingredients that I want to explain a bit more about here, so you know what's important to look for when buying.

MEATS & EGGS

The way animals are raised makes a big difference when it comes to nutrition. If possible, you should always opt for *pasture-raised* pork, chicken, and eggs, and *grass-fed* beef. Meat and eggs from pasture-raised animals retain more nutrients and are raised in a more ethical way than conventionally-raised animals. If you buy grass-fed beef you can be sure that it hasn't been finished with corn or grains, which obviously stay present in the meat. The saying "you are what you eat" definitely applies here, and on the ketogenic diet you don't want your protein sources to be raised on carbs and fillers.

SWEET SUBS

I don't use sweeteners very often, even low-carb ones (my years of strict Paleo got me out of the habit of adding them to my food), but there are some that work well with the keto diet. All-natural *liquid stevia* is good, and in one or two recipes I call for *Swerve*, which is a natural sweetener that measures cup for cup like sugar. However, these ingredients are always optional, so feel free to leave them out.

BUTTER

All fats should come from high-quality sources, whether it's olive oil, coconut oil, or butter. You will notice a lot of my recipes call for butter, which is always a bit of a head-turner when it comes to supposedly "healthy" diets. But as you've learned, fats are a crucial part of what makes keto work. I always keep my refrigerator stocked with lots of high-quality butter made from grass-fed cows. Kerrygold is my favorite brand, and I get the unsalted variety so I can control the salt, depending on what I'm cooking.

WHY THESE FOODS

The 15 foods highlighted in this book have been carefully chosen because they form the building blocks of a solid keto diet. Staying in ketosis relies on a diet of fats, proteins, and vegetables. Staying in ketosis is important because it means your body is continuing to burn fats as energy instead of glucose. People who stay in ketosis are able to lose more weight and often enjoy increased brain function and clarity, better sleep, and decreased appetite overall.

So fats, proteins, and vegetables are what you'll find in these next chapters, and they all work well with a variety of cooking methods. In the first few chapters, we cover the big fats such as eggs, bacon, avocado, dairy, and nuts. We move from there to proteins such as chicken, beef, pork, fish, and seafood. Finally we have five chapters full of recipes based on low-carb veggies such as cabbage, cauliflower, and zucchini. The last chapter is Pantry Basics, and is chock-full of snacks, sauces, and other things you might find yourself making regularly to keep in your refrigerator or pantry.

THE RECIPES

These recipes were developed strategically to help you set up an effective ketogenic diet. You'll find breakfasts, lunches, dinners, snacks, and treats to mix and match to meet your macro goals. Each recipe includes variations that allow you to change up flavors, cooking methods, and macros so you'll never be bored and never have to wonder what you're going to make next.

As I noted previously, you won't encounter any hard-to-find ingredients, and the recipes mostly come together in about 30 minutes. Adopting a new way of eating can be intimidating, even overwhelming, so this book is here to make it as straightforward, manageable, and enjoyable as possible.

Additionally, every recipe and variation includes nutritional calculations including **net carbs**, **total fat**, and **protein** so you can easily monitor your daily allowances and stay on track. For your convenience, the recipes are also labeled:

30 30 Minutes or Fewer	**GF** Gluten-Free
DF Dairy-Free	**NF** Nut-Free

There are many tips included throughout, highlighting ways to make all or part of a recipe ahead, how to make something Paleo, and easy swaps for allergens.

So without further ado, let's get started!

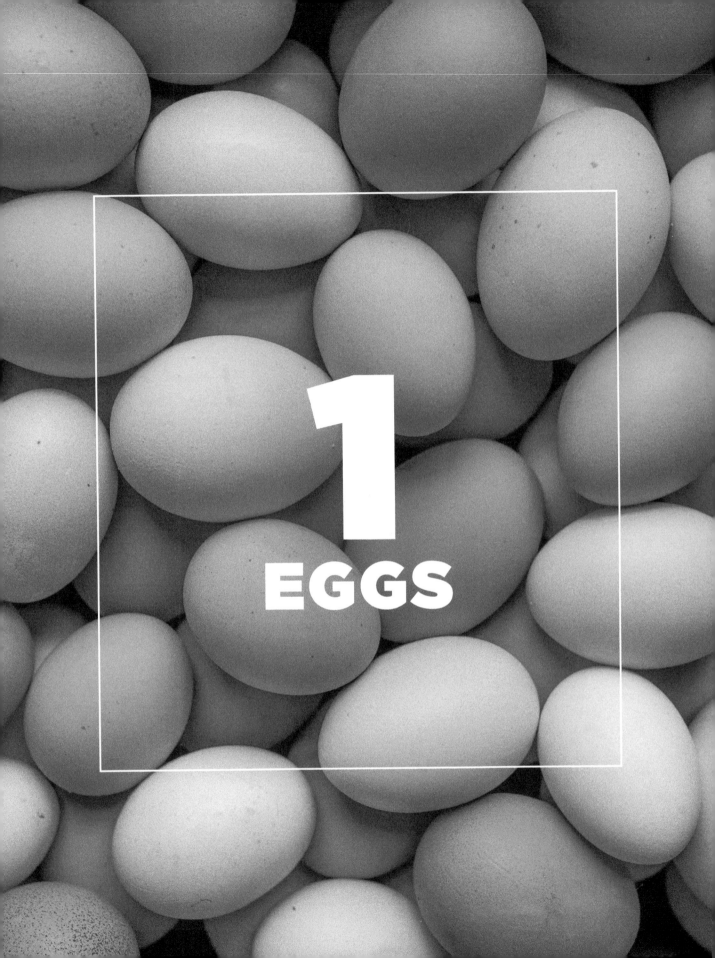

1
EGGS

Eggs are the perfect ingredient to start with because they offer a great way to get protein and fat without many carbs—1 large egg has fewer than 100 calories, 5 grams of fat, about 6 grams of protein, and less than 1 gram of carbohydrates. I like to keep a few hardboiled eggs in the refrigerator so they're always ready to go as a quick snack or into a fast recipe such as my keto Egg Salad (page 11), or even to throw on top of a Cobb Salad (page 81).

A lot of people on the ketogenic diet choose to skip breakfast (intermittent fasting is very interesting, the basic gist being that you fast for 16 hours and eat for 8), but that doesn't mean egg recipes go out the window. Whether you choose to eat breakfast or not, these egg recipes make great lunches, even dinners, and many can be made ahead and eaten as snacks.

I think you'll soon find it's better for your daily macros and meal planning to add some additional fat to your meals (remember: you want to consume more fat than protein) to stay in ketosis, but the following recipes do just that, so you'll stay on the right track!

PERFECT SCRAMBLED EGGS

There are many opinions on how to make the perfect scrambled eggs—and I'm about to add my two cents to the collection. Most people say to cook them *low and slow*; that is, over low heat and very slowly. I personally don't care for the texture that cooking method produces so, over the years, my husband and I have perfected our own recipe—it's *medium-high heat and pretty quickly cooked*, if you will. We make these every weekend and they're great on their own, topped with a little chopped scallion and/or a side of bacon. **MAKES 2 SERVINGS**

PREP TIME: 5 minutes
COOK TIME: 5 minutes

4 eggs

1 to 2 tablespoons water

1 tablespoon butter

Salt

Freshly ground black pepper

Sliced scallion, green parts only, or chopped fresh chives, for topping (optional)

PER SERVING: Calories: 177; Total carbs: 1g; **Net carbs: 1g, 0%;** **Total fat: 15g, 76%; Protein: 11g, 24%;** Fiber: 0g; Sugar: 1g

VARIATION 1: Calories: 190; Total carbs: 1g; **Net carbs: 1g, 0%;** **Total fat: 16g, 76%; Protein: 12g, 24%;** Fiber: 0g; Sugar: 1g

VARIATION 2: Calories: 177; Total carbs: 1g; **Net carbs: 1g, 0%;** **Total fat: 15g, 76%; Protein: 11g, 24%;** Fiber: 0g; Sugar: 1g

ALLERGEN TIP: If you don't tolerate butter, use coconut oil or olive oil instead.

1. Heat a large nonstick skillet over medium-high heat.

2. Into a medium bowl, crack the eggs, add the water, and whisk vigorously until the whites and yolks are well incorporated (you want to be able to lift your whisk from the bowl and have a smooth, continuous strand of egg—nothing lumpy).

3. Add the butter to the skillet and stir with a spatula to coat the entire surface area. Once the butter melts completely, add the eggs and give them a quick stir. Reduce the heat to medium and repeat stirring the eggs and tilting the pan around so the runny parts continue to make contact with the hot surface.

4. When the eggs are mostly cooked, 3 to 4 minutes, reduce the heat to low and continue to fold the eggs over themselves using the spatula.

5. Season with salt and pepper and serve hot when the eggs are cooked to your liking (I prefer mine completely cooked through, but some people like them a little underdone). Top with sliced scallion (if using).

VARIATION 1 **CREAM CHEESE SCRAMBLED EGGS:** To up the fat content of this dish, add 1 tablespoon cream cheese to the pan when the eggs are about two-thirds cooked. Continue to stir until cooked through.

VARIATION 2 **BASIC OMELET:** Instead of stirring the eggs, pour them into the pan and let them cook for a few minutes until the edges are set. If you want, add a few tablespoons of your favorite cheese to the center then carefully fold each side toward the center. Remove from the heat and slide onto a plate to serve.

EGG SALAD

I love making egg salad and keeping it for a few days as a quick lunch or easy snack. Hardboiled eggs are always good to make in batches, but they can get boring on their own, so I sometimes chop them up and toss them with mayo and herbs. Enjoy this egg salad on its own, topping a big salad, or even in a lettuce wrap like a sandwich. It's super easy to customize the flavor and serving methods, which makes this a great recipe to include in your weekly meal plans. **MAKES 4 SERVINGS**

PREP TIME: 15 minutes
COOK TIME: 10 minutes

8 eggs

½ cup Keto Mayonnaise (page 225)

1½ teaspoons yellow mustard

¼ cup chopped scallion, green parts only, or chopped fresh chives

1 tablespoon chopped fresh dill, or 1 teaspoon dried dill

Hot sauce

Salt

Freshly ground black pepper

PER SERVING: Calories: 233; Total carbs: 5g; **Net carbs: 5g, 8%; Total fat: 18g, 70%; Protein: 13g, 22%;** Fiber: 0g; Sugar: 2g

VARIATION 1: Calories: 237; Total carbs: 5g; **Net carbs: 4g, 8%; Total fat: 18g, 70%; Protein: 13g, 22%;** Fiber: 1g; Sugar: 2g

VARIATION 2: Calories: 235; Total carbs: 5g; **Net carbs: 5g, 8%; Total fat: 18g, 70%; Protein: 13g, 22%;** Fiber: 0g; Sugar: 2g

1. In a large saucepan of water that covers the eggs; over high heat, bring the water to a boil. Once the water boils, cover the pan and turn off the heat. Let the pan sit on the warm burner for 8 or 9 minutes. Remove the eggs from the pan and put them in an ice bath to cool. Peel and transfer the eggs to a cutting board.

2. Roughly chop the eggs and transfer them to a large bowl. Add the mayonnaise, mustard, scallion, dill, and a few dashes of hot sauce. Season with salt and pepper. Gently stir to combine. Serve immediately or refrigerate in an airtight container for up to 3 days.

VARIATION 1 **CURRIED EGG SALAD:** Add 1 to 2 teaspoons curry powder to the egg salad for a flavor variation.

VARIATION 2 **LEMON AND DILL EGG SALAD:** Add 2 tablespoons fresh chopped dill and the juice of ½ lemon to the egg salad. Stir well to combine.

MAKE AHEAD: Hardboil the eggs ahead of time so you're one step closer to a fresh batch of egg salad.

DEVILED EGGS

Deviled eggs make a great appetizer, but they're not just for parties. I like to think of them as a fancier way to serve egg salad, since so many of the ingredients are the same (although the flavor does vary a bit and I love the presentation). I always make a lot because leftovers are perfect with a side salad as a quick, keto-friendly lunch, and, of course, you can always pop a couple as a snack at any time. **MAKES 16 DEVILED EGGS**

PREP TIME: 15 minutes
COOK TIME: 20 minutes

8 eggs

½ cup Keto Mayonnaise (page 225)

2 tablespoons pickle relish (not sweet)

1 teaspoon yellow mustard

Salt

Freshly ground black pepper

Paprika, for garnish

PER SERVING (2 deviled eggs): Calories: 178; Total carbs: 2g; **Net carbs: 2g, 3%; Total fat: 16g, 81%; Protein: 7g, 16%;** Fiber: 0g; Sugar: 1g

VARIATION 1: Calories: 331; Total carbs: 2g; **Net carbs: 2g, 1%; Total fat: 28g, 77%; Protein: 18g, 22%;** Fiber: 0g; Sugar: 0g

VARIATION 2: Calories: 178; Total carbs: 2g; **Net carbs: 2g, 3%; Total fat: 16g, 81%; Protein: 7g, 16%;** Fiber: 0g; Sugar 1g

1. Hardboil your eggs using the method from the Egg Salad recipe (see page 11), but let them sit for a full 10 minutes before transferring to the ice bath. Remove the eggs from the ice bath, peel, and halve them lengthwise. Carefully pop the yolks out of the whites into a large bowl. Set the whites aside.

2. To the yolks, add the mayonnaise, relish, and mustard. Season with salt and pepper. Mix well with a fork until all the ingredients are thoroughly combined and the mixture has a smooth consistency.

3. Carefully spoon the yolk filling into each hardboiled egg white half and garnish with a sprinkle of paprika.

VARIATION 1 **BACON DEVILED EGGS:** Top each deviled egg with a small (1-ounce) piece of cooked bacon.

VARIATION 2 **PIPED DEVILED EGGS:** Instead of spooning the filling into the egg whites, transfer the yolk mixture to a large freezer bag. Twist the bag tightly, cut the tip off like a piping bag, and pipe the filling into each egg white. It's an extra step but I think it makes filling the eggs a lot easier, plus it looks prettier.

KETO EGG "MCMUFFINS"

One of the hardest parts of adopting a new diet lifestyle is letting go of those old guilty pleasures. For me, that's the egg sandwich—more specifically, the Egg McMuffin. Let's get real: English muffins are delicious. But they aren't low-carb, so that's where this recipe steps in. We cook the eggs into perfect little circles and use them as the "bread" in this sausage and cheese sandwich, so it has almost the same look of those perfect-every-time fast-food breakfast sandwiches, but without the carbs. **MAKES 2 SANDWICHES**

PREP TIME: 5 minutes
COOK TIME: 10 minutes

1 tablespoon butter

4 eggs

2 cooked breakfast sausage patties

2 slices Cheddar cheese

Salt

Freshly ground black pepper

PER SERVING (1 sandwich):
Calories: 397; Total carbs: 1g;
**Net carbs: 1g, 0%; Total fat: 34g, 77%;
Protein: 23g, 23%;** Fiber: 0g; Sugar: 1g

VARIATION 1: Calories: 495;
Total carbs: 1g; **Net carbs: 1g, 0%;
Total fat: 40g, 73%; Protein: 32g, 27%;**
Fiber: 0g; Sugar: 1g

VARIATION 2: Calories: 397;
Total carbs: 1g; **Net carbs: 1g, 0%;
Total fat: 34g, 77%; Protein: 23g, 23%;**
Fiber: 0g; Sugar: 1g

1. Heat a large nonstick skillet over medium heat. Add the butter and let it melt.

2. Crack each egg into a round metal biscuit cutter, silicone mold, or just the ring of a mason jar lid, and give it a quick stir as it cooks, gently breaking the yolk. Cook for 3 to 4 minutes or until set. Remove from the mold. Repeat until all the eggs are cooked.

3. In the same skillet, heat the sausage for 1 to 2 minutes to warm. Top each piece with 1 slice of cheese. You can cover the skillet to help the cheese melt more quickly.

4. Assemble the sandwiches by placing a cheesy sausage on 1 egg and topping it with a second egg. Repeat with the remaining sandwich ingredients and serve immediately.

VARIATION 1 **BACON EGG AND CHEESE SANDWICHES:** Swap out the sausage for a few pieces of bacon. You can melt the cheese directly onto one of the eggs, top with bacon, add the other egg, and serve.

VARIATION 2 **KETO EGG "MCMUFFINS" OVER MEDIUM:** If you like your egg sandwiches a little runny, leave the yolk intact and cook for only about 2 minutes, just until the whites are set.

MAKE AHEAD: Make a big batch of eggs ahead of time (2 or 3 days at most) and refrigerate until ready to serve (this would be perfect for a big breakfast party or just to make your weekday mornings easier). Reheat in a 350°F oven for 15 to 20 minutes until warmed through.

SANTA FE FRITTATA

I love making frittatas for breakfast when I have people over—they're easy to make; nice and big so you can feed a ton of people, and I usually have a little left over, which makes for a nice lunch later on. But oftentimes I end up throwing the same old thing into it. This Santa Fe Frittata is fun because it incorporates pork sausage and veggies with pepper jack cheese—although I have to say my favorite part is the sour cream on top, so don't forget it! **MAKES 4 SERVINGS**

PREP TIME: 10 minutes
COOK TIME: 30 minutes

1 to 2 tablespoons olive oil

½ onion, diced

2 garlic cloves, minced

6 ounces ground pork sausage

½ red bell pepper, diced

½ green bell pepper, diced

Salt

Freshly ground black pepper

6 eggs

½ cup shredded pepper jack cheese

Sliced scallion, for garnish

Salsa, for garnish

Sour cream, for garnish

Fresh cilantro leaves, for garnish

PER SERVING: Calories: 493;
Total carbs: 4g; **Net carbs: 3g, 3%;**
Total fat: 41g, 75%; Protein: 27g, 22%;
Fiber: 1g; Sugar: 2g

VARIATION 1: Calories: 535;
Total carbs: 5g; **Net carbs: 4g, 4%;**
Total fat: 43g, 72%; Protein: 32g, 24%;
Fiber: 1g; Sugar: 2g

VARIATION 2: Calories: 493;
Total carbs: 4g; **Net carbs: 3g, 3%;**
Total fat: 41g, 75%; Protein: 27g, 22%;
Fiber: 1g; Sugar: 2g

1. Preheat the oven to 350°F.

2. In a cast-iron skillet over medium heat, heat the olive oil.

3. Add the onion and garlic. Sauté for 5 to 7 minutes until the onion is softened and translucent.

4. Add the sausage. Cook for 5 to 7 minutes or until browned, stirring to break up the meat.

5. Add the red and green bell peppers and stir gently. Season with salt and pepper.

6. In a large bowl, whisk the eggs. Arrange the onion, sausage, and pepper mixture in the skillet so the ingredients are evenly distributed. Slowly pour the eggs over the top. Increase the heat to medium high. Season with salt and pepper and cook for 3 to 4 minutes until the edges start to pull away from the skillet.

7. Top the frittata with cheese and transfer to the oven. Cook for 15 to 20 minutes until the top is no longer runny. Remove from the oven, cool slightly, and serve garnished with scallion, salsa, sour cream, and a few cilantro leaves.

8. Refrigerate leftovers in an airtight container for up to 3 days.

VARIATION 1 **DENVER FRITTATA:** Switch the pepper jack cheese to Cheddar and add 3 to 4 ounces diced cooked ham to the egg mixture before baking. Top with salsa and sour cream or another sprinkle of Cheddar.

VARIATION 2 **STOVE TOP FRITTATA:** Cook the frittata completely on the stove top and skip the oven heat; just cover the pan at step 7 and cook until the eggs are completely set.

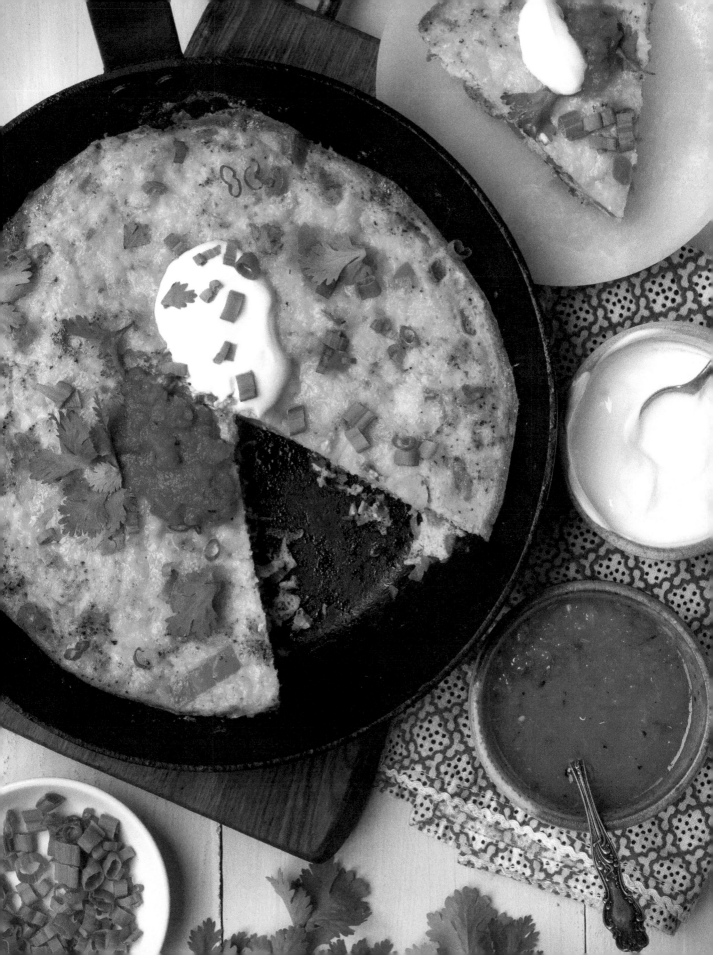

BACON AND EGG CUPS

Bacon, eggs, a little salt and pepper—the perfect breakfast or snack is just a few ingredients away! I like to precook the bacon a bit to reduce the baking time, but if you have an extra 10 to 15 minutes, do it all in the oven. These bacon and egg cups make a lovely, really easy breakfast. **MAKES 6 SERVINGS**

PREP TIME: 10 minutes
COOK TIME: 25 minutes

Nonstick cooking spray

6 bacon slices

6 eggs

Salt

Freshly ground black pepper

Sliced scallion, green parts only, for garnish (optional)

PER SERVING: Calories: 164;
Total carbs: 1g; **Net carbs: 1g, 0%;**
Total fat: 12g, 68%; Protein: 13g, 32%;
Fiber: 0g; Sugar: 0g

VARIATION 1: Calories: 282;
Total carbs: 1g; **Net carbs: 1g, 0%;**
Total fat: 22g, 70%; Protein: 20g, 30%;
Fiber: 0g; Sugar: 1g

VARIATION 2: Calories: 204;
Total carbs: **2g; Net carbs: 1g, 3%;**
Total fat: 16g, 71%; Protein: 13g, 26%;
Fiber: 1g; Sugar: 0g

1. Preheat the oven to 350°F.

2. Lightly coat the wells of a muffin pan with cooking spray.

3. In a medium skillet over medium heat, lightly cook the bacon for about 5 minutes. You aren't fully cooking it or even getting it crispy, just closer to being done (and still bendable). Transfer the bacon to a paper towel-lined plate to drain.

4. Line each well of the muffin pan with 1 bacon slice around the bottom edge. Crack 1 egg into each cup and season with salt and pepper.

5. Bake for about 20 minutes or until the whites are set and the yolks are cooked to your liking. Top with sliced scallion (if using) and serve.

VARIATION 1 **BACON EGG AND CHEESE CUPS:** Add ½ to 1 ounce shredded cheese on top of each egg for some extra fat and cheesy goodness.

VARIATION 2 **BACON AND EGG CUPS WITH AVOCADO:** Dice ½ avocado and add a few pieces to each bacon and egg cup before baking.

BAKED EGGS IN AVOCADO

These baked eggs in avocado are a great weekday breakfast you can make quickly before heading out the door. Like a lot of the recipes in this cookbook, this one calls for minimal ingredients and fewer than 30 minutes of your time. All you do is cut an avocado, scoop some out, and crack in your eggs! Preheat the oven while you're making your morning coffee and you'll have breakfast before you know it. **MAKES 2 SERVINGS**

PREP TIME: 5 minutes
COOK TIME: 15 to 20 minutes

1 ripe avocado, halved and pitted

2 eggs

Salt

Freshly ground black pepper

Hot sauce (optional)

PER SERVING: Calories: 275; Total carbs: 9g; **Net carbs: 2g, 13%; Total fat: 23g, 75%; Protein: 8g, 12%;** Fiber: 7g; Sugar: 1g

VARIATION 1: Calories: 314; Total carbs: 10g; **Net carbs: 3g, 13%; Total fat: 26g, 74%; Protein: 10g, 13%;** Fiber: 7g; Sugar: 1g

VARIATION 2: Calories: 279; Total carbs: 10g; **Net carbs: 3g, 14%; Total fat: 23g, 74%; Protein: 8g, 12%;** Fiber: 7g; Sugar: 1g

1. Preheat the oven to 425°F.

2. Scoop out 1 or 2 tablespoons of avocado flesh from each half and set aside for another recipe (see 3. Avocado, page 35, for lots of ideas). Place the scooped avocado halves in a small baking dish.

3. Carefully crack 1 egg into each half. Season with salt and pepper.

4. Bake for 15 to 20 minutes or until the whites are set and the yolks are cooked to your liking. Sprinkle with some hot sauce (if using) and serve immediately.

VARIATION 1 **GARLIC PARMESAN BAKED EGGS IN AVOCADO:** Follow the recipe as written, but season the eggs in the avocado halves with about 1 teaspoon garlic powder. Top each with 1 tablespoon grated Parmesan cheese and bake according to the instructions.

VARIATION 2 **SALSA LIME BAKED EGGS IN AVOCADO:** Follow the recipe as written, but top each finished avocado with 1 tablespoon of your favorite salsa and a sprinkling of freshly squeezed lime juice.

BAKED EGGS FLORENTINE

My mom and I used to go to this little bakery in Roanoke, Virginia, for breakfast. We'd split a French press and both order the eggs Florentine, which came in a lovely one-person casserole dish with perfectly baked eggs nestled within delicious, bubbling, melty cheese and creamed spinach. They would serve it with some toasty slices from a baguette, but I swear it was just as good without the bread. **MAKES 2 SERVINGS**

PREP TIME: 15 minutes
COOK TIME: 30 minutes

10 ounces fresh spinach

2 tablespoons butter

¼ white onion, diced

2 garlic cloves, minced

Salt

Freshly ground black pepper

¼ cup heavy (whipping) cream

2 ounces shredded Parmesan cheese, divided

4 eggs

2 ounces crumbled feta cheese

PER SERVING: Calories: 502;
Total carbs: 11g; **Net carbs: 7g, 9%;**
Total fat: 38g, 68%; Protein: 29g, 23%;
Fiber: 4g; Sugar: 3g

VARIATION 1: Calories: 633;
Total carbs: 11g; **Net carbs: 7g, 7%;**
Total fat: 45g, 64%; Protein: 46g, 29%;
Fiber: 4g; Sugar: 3g

VARIATION 2: Calories: 506;
Total carbs: 12g; **Net carbs: 8g, 9%;**
Total fat: 38g, 68%; Protein: 29g, 23%;
Fiber: 4g; Sugar: 4g

1. Preheat the oven to 400°F.

2. In a large pan over medium-low heat, wilt the spinach slightly for 4 to 5 minutes. Transfer the spinach to a colander and rinse with cool water. With your hands or in paper towels, squeeze the spinach to drain as much water as possible from it. Transfer to a cutting board and chop.

3. In the same pan over medium heat, melt the butter.

4. Add the onion and garlic. Sauté for 5 to 7 minutes until the onion is softened and translucent.

5. Return the spinach to the pan and season well with salt and pepper.

6. Add the heavy cream and 1 ounce of Parmesan. Reduce the heat to medium low and continue to cook for 3 to 4 minutes more or until everything is well combined. Transfer the creamed spinach to two small (9-inch diameter) baking dishes; if you don't have these, put the spinach in one dish and divide it when serving.

7. Use a spoon to create small hollows, or nests, for the eggs. Crack 2 eggs into each dish. Top with the feta and remaining 1 ounce of Parmesan cheese, seasoning with a bit more salt and pepper. Bake for 15 to 20 minutes or until the egg whites are set but the yolks are still a bit runny.

VARIATION 1 **BAKED EGGS FLORENTINE WITH PROSCIUTTO:**
Add about 2 ounces sliced prosciutto to each baking dish and
follow the rest of the recipe as written.

VARIATION 2 **BAKED EGGS FLORENTINE WITH TOMATO:**
Before these go into the oven, top each dish with 1 to 2 ounces
diced fresh tomato and another sprinkle of shredded
Parmesan cheese.

MAKE AHEAD: Prepare the creamed spinach ahead of time and keep it
refrigerated. Assemble everything and pop the dishes in the oven 20 to
30 minutes before you're ready to serve.

ALMOND FLOUR TORTILLAS

I started making these almond flour tortillas a few years ago when I was searching for a great Paleo (and low-carb) substitute. I originally made a more pancake-style version with eggs and almond flour and some cinnamon, but I thought it would be really good with savory spices instead. These tortillas keep well in the refrigerator for several days and are sturdy enough to hold whatever you might dream of wrapping them around. **MAKES 5 TORTILLAS**

PREP TIME: 10 minutes
COOK TIME: 25 minutes

10 eggs

6 tablespoons almond flour

3 tablespoons arrowroot powder

1 teaspoon garlic powder

Salt

Freshly ground black pepper

2 to 3 tablespoons butter, divided

PER SERVING (1 tortilla):
Calories: 225; Total carbs: 6g;
Net carbs: 6g, 11%; Total fat: 17g, 68%;
Protein: 12g, 21%; Fiber: 0g; Sugar: 1g

VARIATION 1: Calories: 486;
Total carbs: 10g; **Net carbs: 9g, 8%;**
Total fat: 34g, 63%; Protein: 35g, 29%;
Fiber: 1g; Sugar: 3g

VARIATION 2: Calories: 226;
Total carbs: 6g; **Net carbs: 5g, 11%;**
Total fat: 17g, 68%; Protein: 12g, 21%;
Fiber: 1g; Sugar: 1g

1. Heat a large skillet over medium-high heat.

2. In a large bowl whisk the eggs.

3. Sift the almond flour and arrowroot powder into the bowl and add the garlic powder. Season with salt and pepper.

4. Add 1 tablespoon of butter to the skillet to melt. Pour in about ¼ cup of the batter. Tilt the skillet around so the batter evenly coats the bottom. Cook for 2 to 3 minutes or until the edges begin to pull away from the skillet. Use a spatula to flip the tortilla and let it cook on the other side for 1 to 2 minutes. Transfer to a plate and repeat, adding a bit more butter and another ¼ cup of batter until the ingredients have been used up. Serve immediately.

VARIATION 1 **TURKEY CLUB WRAPS:** Fill with 2 ounces sliced turkey, 1 cooked bacon slice, chopped lettuce, 1 or 2 tomato slices, 1 piece Monterey Jack cheese, and 1 tablespoon Keto Mayonnaise (page 225).

VARIATION 2 **SWEET TORTILLAS:** Substitute cinnamon for the garlic powder and add 1 teaspoon vanilla extract (if you'd like—and can swing the carbs—you could add a little bit of stevia to sweeten the batter). Follow the rest of the recipe as written and serve with butter and/or a few chopped fresh raspberries.

LOW-CARB EGG CURRY

This egg curry is a great low-carb vegetarian dish, which can sometimes be hard to find when you're eating a keto diet. It's a nice variation on regular hard-boiled eggs, which can become pretty boring if you eat them often enough. This curry recipe marinates hardboiled eggs in a delicious, spicy sauce that comes together a lot faster than traditional curries. You can also make it ahead of time and keep it in the refrigerator until needed. **MAKES 4 SERVINGS**

PREP TIME: 15 minutes
COOK TIME: 20 minutes

  NF

½ onion, finely diced

1 small (1-inch) knob fresh ginger

2 garlic cloves

1 small green chile pepper

1 large Roma tomato

1 tablespoon ghee

2 teaspoons ground turmeric

2 teaspoons chili powder

2 teaspoons ground coriander

2 teaspoons garam masala

½ cup water

Salt

Freshly ground black pepper

4 hardboiled eggs, peeled (see page 11)

PER SERVING: Calories: 128; Total carbs: 7g; **Net carbs: 5g, 22%;** **Total fat: 8g, 56%; Protein: 7g, 22%;** Fiber: 2g; Sugar: 2g

VARIATION 1: Calories: 210; Total carbs: 7g; **Net carbs: 5g, 13%;** **Total fat: 14g, 60%; Protein: 14g, 27%;** Fiber: 2g; Sugar: 2g

VARIATION 2: Calories: 177; Total carbs: 8g; **Net carbs: 6g, 18%;** **Total fat: 13g, 66%; Protein: 7g, 16%;** Fiber: 2g; Sugar: 2g

1. In a food processor or blender, combine the onion, ginger, garlic, and chile pepper. Process until a paste forms. Transfer to a small bowl and set aside.

2. Rinse out the blender then purée the tomato in it. Set aside.

3. In a small saucepan over medium heat, melt the ghee. Add the onion-ginger-garlic-chile paste to the pan. Stir and let it cook for 3 to 4 minutes or until fragrant.

4. Stir in the turmeric, chili powder, coriander, and garam masala.

5. Stir in the puréed tomato. Cook for 1 to 2 minutes then add the water, stirring to thoroughly combine. Season with salt and pepper, cover the pan, and cook for about 10 minutes over low heat.

6. Add the peeled eggs to the curry and gently stir to get all sides coated with the sauce. Cook for 3 to 5 minutes over low heat and serve.

VARIATION 1 **LOW-CARB CHICKEN CURRY:** Instead of eggs, serve this curry over 4 to 6 ounces cooked chicken (grill chicken thighs before or while you make the curry—see Easy Marinated Chicken Thighs, page 89).

VARIATION 2 **CREAMY EGG CURRY:** Make this more of a cream-based sauce by adding ½ cup heavy (whipping) cream instead of water.

PERFECT PAIR: Serve with Cauliflower Rice (page 178).

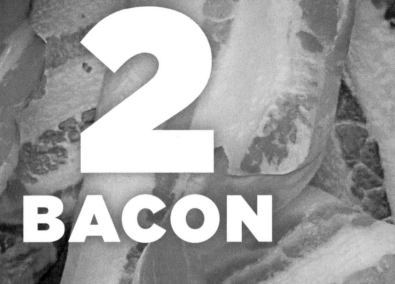

2
BACON

Bacon really had its moment a few years ago—you could get bacon on your Bloody Mary, bacon cupcakes, bacon beer—you name it, there was bacon in it. The fad may be on its way out, but bacon is still a keto staple because it's a great way to get both protein and fat, and you can easily make it either the center of a recipe or just a supporting ingredient.

I like making a big batch in the oven on Sunday and using it in recipes throughout the week, whether on a salad, as a side with scrambled eggs, or in any of the following recipes where it plays a larger part. Over the next few pages you'll find appetizers, main dishes, dips, soups, and easy lunch ideas and they all have one thing in common: bacon.

A note about ingredients: Carefully read the labels on your bacon packages. Many brands have a lot of added sugar. You want as few ingredients as possible in your bacon, and double-check the nutritional info before you buy it to make sure it's not full of unnecessary carbohydrates.

BACON RANCH DIP

It was dishes like this one that made me fall in love with keto. I am a self-professed lover of carbs, but I never really feel deprived when there are super-rich, decadent, and absolutely satisfying recipes to enjoy. This dip is a great dish to bring to a party or just to make at home and dip veggies into whenever you need a snack. **MAKES ABOUT 10 SERVINGS**

PREP TIME: 10 minutes
COOK TIME: 10 minutes

1 (8-ounce) package full-fat cream cheese, at room temperature

1 cup full-fat sour cream

8 bacon slices, cooked and crumbled

1½ teaspoons dried chives

1 teaspoon dry mustard

½ teaspoon dried dill

½ teaspoon celery seed

½ teaspoon garlic powder

½ teaspoon onion powder

Salt

Freshly ground black pepper

¼ cup sliced scallion, or fresh chives, for garnish

PER SERVING: Calories: 211; Total carbs: 2g; **Net carbs: 2g, 4%;** **Total fat: 19g, 81%; Protein: 8g, 15%;** Fiber: 0g; Sugar: 0g

VARIATION 1: Calories: 228; Total carbs: 3g; **Net carbs: 3g, 5%;** **Total fat: 20g, 79%; Protein: 9g, 16%;** Fiber: 0g; Sugar: 0g

VARIATION 2: Calories: 211; Total carbs: 2g; **Net carbs: 2g, 4%;** **Total fat: 19g, 81%; Protein: 8g, 15%;** Fiber: 0g; Sugar: 0g

1. In a medium bowl, stir the cream cheese until it becomes fluffy and smooth. Add the sour cream and gently fold to combine.

2. Add the bacon, chives, mustard, dill, celery seed, garlic powder, and onion powder. Season with salt and pepper and stir to combine. Top with the scallion and serve immediately, or refrigerate in an airtight container for up to 1 week.

VARIATION 1 **BACON CHEDDAR RANCH DIP:** Add 1 cup shredded Cheddar cheese to the mix and stir well to combine.

VARIATION 2 **BUFFALO BACON RANCH DIP:** Add ½ cup Frank's RedHot Sauce to the mix and stir well to combine. Add more if you like it spicier.

MAKE AHEAD: Make this dip 1 day before you plan to serve it. If you don't feel like gathering all the spices, use a package or two of dried ranch dressing mix.

BACON-WRAPPED CHEESE BITES

These bacon-wrapped cheese bites are a keto take on the classic mozzarella stick. Instead of battering them in flour, here they are wrapped in bacon for a nice crunch. These are best right out of the skillet, all hot bacon and melty cheese, but if you want to make them ahead and reheat all or some of them quickly in the oven, you could totally do that as well. **MAKES ABOUT 36 BITES**

PREP TIME: 15 minutes
COOK TIME: 10 minutes

1 package (usually 12 pieces) string cheese, or mozzarella sticks, cut widthwise into thirds

1 (1-pound) package keto-friendly bacon, halved widthwise

PER SERVING (2 bites):
Calories: 175; Total carbs: 1g;
Net carbs: 1g, 2%; Total fat: 15g, 77%;
Protein: 9g, 21%; Fiber: 0g; Sugar: 0g

VARIATION 1: Calories: 175;
Total carbs: 1g; **Net carbs: 1g, 2%;**
Total fat: 15g, 77%; Protein: 9g, 21%;
Fiber: 0g; Sugar: 0g

VARIATION 2: Calories: 68;
Total carbs: 2g; **Net carbs: 1g, 18%;**
Total fat: 4g, 47%; Protein: 6g, 35%;
Fiber: 1g; Sugar: 1g

1. Wrap 1 piece of bacon lengthwise around a piece of cheese. Wrap another piece of bacon widthwise around the cheese so the entire piece of cheese is covered with bacon. Repeat with the remaining cheese and bacon pieces.

2. In a large nonstick skillet over medium-high heat, cook the bacon-wrapped cheese bites for 2 to 3 minutes per side or until the bacon is cooked through and crisp. Remove from the heat and serve.

VARIATION 1 **OVEN-BAKED BACON-WRAPPED CHEESE BITES:** Instead of panfrying these, space them evenly on a baking sheet and bake at 425°F for 15 to 20 minutes until the bacon is cooked, flipping once halfway through the cooking time.

VARIATION 2 **JALAPEÑO-WRAPPED CHEESE BITES:** Instead of bacon, use a hollowed-out jalapeño pepper to wrap the cheese. Bake at 375°F for 15 to 20 minutes until the peppers are slightly softened.

PERFECT PAIR: Serve with a side of Ranch Dressing (page 225) for dipping.

BACON BRUSSELS SPROUTS

These Brussels sprouts are my go-to side dish whenever I want something delicious but easy. My whole family enjoys them and I try to make them whenever we gather together for any kind of potluck lunch or dinner. My husband and I absolutely love really crispy Brussels sprouts and always order them any time we see them on a menu; we have an ongoing collection of favorites, but (happily) my own recipe has managed to stay on the list. **MAKES 4 SERVINGS**

PREP TIME: 5 minutes
COOK TIME: 20 minutes

2 bacon slices

2 cups Brussels sprouts, halved

Salt

Freshly ground black pepper

1 tablespoon butter

PER SERVING: Calories: 99;
Total carbs: 4g; **Net carbs: 2g, 16%;**
Total fat: 7g, 64%; Protein: 5g, 20%;
Fiber: 2g; Sugar: 1g

VARIATION 1: Calories: 109;
Total carbs: 5g; **Net carbs: 3g, 18%;**
Total fat: 9g, 74%; Protein: 2g, 8%;
Fiber: 2g; Sugar: 1g

VARIATION 2: Calories: 99;
Total carbs: 4g; **Net carbs: 2g, 16%;**
Total fat: 7g, 64%; Protein: 5g, 20%;
Fiber: 2g; Sugar: 1g

1. In a large skillet over medium-high heat, cook the bacon for about 5 minutes or until crispy. Transfer to a paper towel-lined plate to drain; leave the bacon fat in the skillet.

2. Add the Brussels sprouts to the hot bacon fat in the skillet. Cook over medium-high heat for about 15 minutes until they get golden brown and crispy. Season with salt and pepper.

3. Add the butter and cook for 2 to 3 minutes more, stirring occasionally to prevent burning.

4. While the Brussels sprouts cook, cut the bacon into bite-size pieces. Serve the sprouts hot, topped with the bacon.

VARIATION 1 **BUFFALO BRUSSELS SPROUTS:** Skip the bacon and cook the Brussels sprouts in 3 tablespoons butter, tossing them in ½ cup Frank's RedHot Sauce once they're nice and crispy.

VARIATION 2 **OVEN-ROASTED BRUSSELS SPROUTS:** Place Brussels sprouts in an even layer on a large rimmed baking sheet. Pour 2 to 3 tablespoons olive oil over them and mix well with your hands to combine. Add chopped raw bacon and continue to stir. Season with salt and pepper and bake at 375°F for 20 to 30 minutes or until the sprouts have browned and the edges are beginning to crisp.

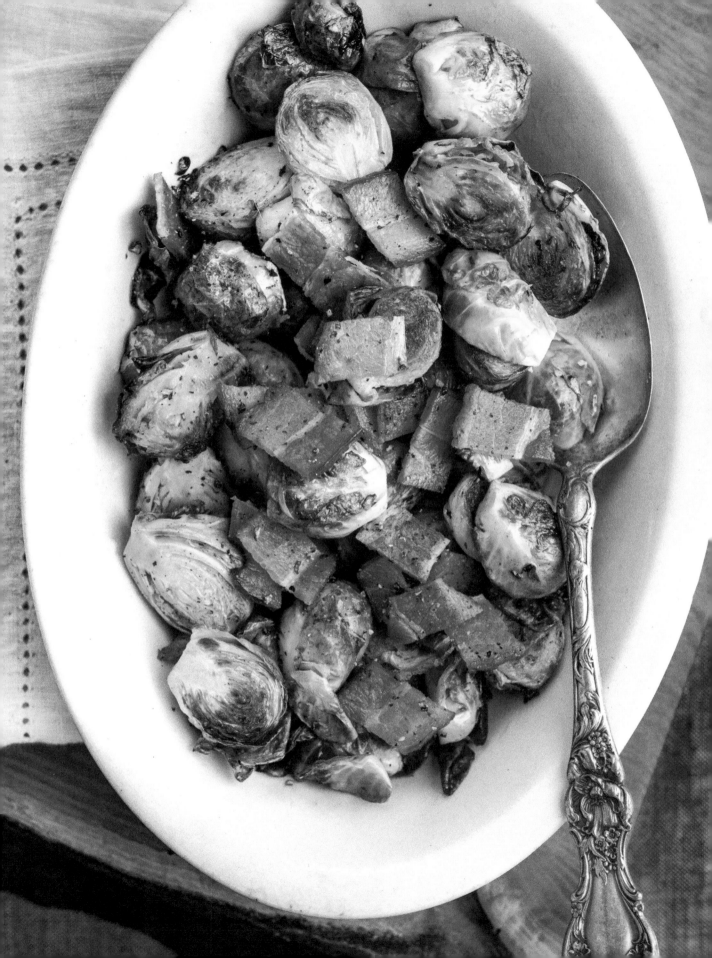

BACON-WRAPPED SCALLOPS

My brother makes the best scallops—he usually seasons them heavily and sears them in a super-hot pan. He was my inspiration for these bacon-wrapped scallops, although I bake them and serve them as an appetizer. Scallops are great because they cook really fast, and I love their lightness and texture when combined with smoky bacon. **MAKES 4 SERVINGS**

PREP TIME: 10 minutes
COOK TIME: 15 minutes

2 tablespoons butter, melted, plus more for the baking sheet

1 pound scallops, rinsed under cold water and patted dry with a paper towel

1 (1-pound) package keto-friendly bacon, slices halved widthwise

Salt

Freshly ground black pepper

PER SERVING: Calories: 599; Total carbs: 2g; **Net carbs: 2g, 1%; Total fat: 51g, 77%; Protein: 33g, 22%;** Fiber: 0g; Sugar: 0g

VARIATION 1: Calories: 599; Total carbs: 2g; **Net carbs: 2g, 1%; Total fat: 51g, 77%; Protein: 33g, 22%;** Fiber: 0g; Sugar: 0g

VARIATION 2: Calories: 615; Total carbs: 1g; **Net carbs: 1g, 0%; Total fat: 51g, 75%; Protein: 38g, 25%;** Fiber: 0g; Sugar: 0g

1. Preheat the oven to 425°F.

2. Lightly grease a rimmed baking sheet with butter or olive oil.

3. Wrap each scallop with 1 half piece of bacon. Secure with a toothpick.

4. Brush the top of each scallop with melted butter and season with salt and pepper. Place on the prepared sheet and bake for 15 to 20 minutes, flipping halfway through the cooking time, until the scallops are opaque and the bacon is on the crispy side.

VARIATION 1 **SMOKED PAPRIKA BACON-WRAPPED SCALLOPS:** For a smokier flavor, season the scallops with a sprinkle of smoked paprika before baking.

VARIATION 2 **BACON-WRAPPED SHRIMP:** Instead of scallops, use 1 pound large (peeled) shrimp with the tails still on. Panfry for 3 to 4 minutes per side, or bake as directed in the recipe.

BACON-WRAPPED CHEESE DOGS

Hot dogs are kind of a backup-plan dinner in our house—we always have them in the refrigerator and can throw them on the grill when we don't have anything planned but don't want to go out or splurge for high-carb delivery (usually Chinese food). After a few basic hot dog dinners, we started adding cheese and bacon to liven them up. Is there anything better than a cheesy hot dog with bacon? **MAKES 8 DOGS**

PREP TIME: 5 minutes
COOK TIME: 10 minutes

  NF

4 slices Cheddar cheese, cut into strips about the width of each hot dog (or about ½ cup shredded)

8 all-beef hot dogs, halved lengthwise

8 bacon slices

PER SERVING (2 dogs): Calories: 762; Total carbs: 4g; **Net carbs: 4g, 2%;** **Total fat: 66g, 78%; Protein: 38g, 20%;** Fiber: 0g; Sugar: 4g

VARIATION 1: Calories: 562; Total carbs: 4g; **Net carbs: 4g, 3%;** **Total fat: 50g, 80%; Protein: 24g, 17%;** Fiber: 0g; Sugar: 4g

VARIATION 2: Calories: 762; Total carbs: 4g; **Net carbs: 4g, 2%;** **Total fat: 66g, 78%; Protein: 38g, 20%;** Fiber: 0g; Sugar: 4g

1. Layer cheese strips onto the bottom half of each dog. Top with the other half.

2. Wrap each hot dog in 1 bacon slice. Place the bacon-wrapped cheese dogs in a large skillet, or on the grill, over medium-high heat. Let the bacon cook on all sides, 7 to 10 minutes total. Refrigerate leftovers in an airtight container for up to 1 week. Reheat in the microwave for 30 seconds to 1 minute.

VARIATION 1 **JALAPEÑO-WRAPPED CHEESE DOGS:** Skip the bacon and use a jalapeño to hold these dogs together if you're in the mood for something spicy—just cut the top and bottom off each pepper and remove the seeds. Slide it over the cheese-filled dog. Cook as directed, or see the oven-baked variation.

VARIATION 2 **OVEN-BAKED BACON-WRAPPED CHEESE DOGS:** Instead of a skillet, cook these hot dogs in the oven at 375°F for about 15 to 20 minutes or until the bacon is cooked through and crispy.

PERFECT PAIR: Serve these dogs with a side of Low-Carb Ketchup (page 226).

BLT WRAPS

This is one of the easiest lunches in the world. It's basically a BLT, but using a romaine lettuce leaf as a wrap instead of bread. The combination of bacon, lettuce, tomato, and (lots of) mayo is one of my favorites—I have it (or something similar) for lunch at least once a week! **MAKES 2 WRAPS**

PREP TIME: 10 minutes
COOK TIME: 0 minutes

4 bacon slices, cooked

2 large romaine lettuce leaves, washed and dried

4 pieces thinly sliced tomato

2 tablespoons Keto Mayonnaise (page 225)

PER SERVING (1 wrap): Calories: 251; Total carbs: 5g; **Net carbs: 4g, 8%;** **Total fat: 19g, 68%; Protein: 15g, 24%;** Fiber: 1g; Sugar: 3g

VARIATION 1: Calories: 332; Total carbs: 8g; **Net carbs: 6g, 10%;** **Total fat: 20g, 54%; Protein: 30g, 36%;** Fiber: 2g; Sugar: 6g

VARIATION 2: Calories: 260; Total carbs: 5g; **Net carbs: 4g, 8%;** **Total fat: 20g, 69%; Protein: 15g, 23%;** Fiber: 1g; Sugar: 2g

If needed, slightly reheat the bacon in the microwave for 20 to 30 seconds. Assemble the wraps: Place 2 bacon slices on each lettuce leaf. Top each with 2 tomato slices and 1 tablespoon of mayonnaise. Wrap up or fold over and serve immediately.

VARIATION 1 **TURKEY BLT WRAPS:** Add 2 slices of your favorite deli turkey to each wrap.

VARIATION 2 **BLT SALAD:** Instead of a wrap, serve this as a salad: Chop the lettuce (add a few more leaves) and top with crumbled bacon and diced tomato. Serve with Ranch Dressing (page 225) instead of the mayo.

BACON AVOCADO MOUSSE CUPS

I picked up premade guacamole from the store a while ago and was surprised to see it had Greek yogurt in it. I didn't think I would like it, but it ended up being so good it inspired this whole recipe! These mousse cups are really delicious and super cute—you just bake the bacon into cups using a mini muffin pan then fill them with a tangy avocado mousse packed with lots of flavor.

MAKES 6 SERVINGS

PREP TIME: 10 minutes
COOK TIME: 20 minutes

12 bacon slices

2 or 3 ripe avocados, halved and pitted

½ cup plain Greek yogurt

Juice of ½ lime

Salt

Freshly ground black pepper

PER SERVING (2 filled cups): Calories: 530; Total carbs: 16g; **Net carbs: 9g, 12%; Total fat: 38g, 65%; Protein: 31g, 23%;** Fiber: 7g; Sugar: 5g

VARIATION 1: Calories: 468; Total carbs: 10g; **Net carbs: 3g, 8%; Total fat: 40g, 77%; Protein: 17g, 15%;** Fiber: 7g; Sugar: 1g

VARIATION 2: Calories: 532; Total carbs: 16g; **Net carbs: 9g, 12%; Total fat: 38g, 65%; Protein: 31g, 23%;** Fiber: 7g: Sugar: 5g

1. Preheat the oven to 425°F.

2. Wrap each piece of bacon around the sides and bottom of the wells of a mini muffin tin to create little bacon cups. Bake for 15 to 20 minutes or until the bacon is cooked through and crisp.

3. While the bacon cooks, in a medium bowl, combine the avocado flesh, yogurt, and lime juice. Mix well until combined and smooth. Season with salt and pepper and transfer to a piping bag (or a plastic bag with the tip cut off).

4. Remove the bacon from the oven and cool slightly. Pipe each bacon cup full of avocado mousse. Serve immediately.

VARIATION 1 **BACON AVOCADO MOUSSE CUPS WITH SOUR CREAM:** Swap in sour cream for the Greek yogurt.

VARIATION 2 **BACON AVOCADO MOUSSE CUPS WITH MUSTARD:** Add 1 tablespoon grainy Dijon mustard to the avocado mousse for a nice flavor variation.

MAKE IT PALEO: Skip the yogurt and fill with Everyday Guacamole (page 38). Top with chopped fresh cilantro.

TURKEY CLUB PINWHEELS

I have always loved turkey club sandwiches—I still do! I remember as a kid ordering them for breakfast or lunch after church on Sundays with my family. These turkey club pinwheels have all the same ingredients, but instead of sliced bread, they're held together with a keto-friendly wrap. I use my Almond Flour Tortillas (page 20); if you tolerate wheat, look for good low-carb tortillas at the store. **MAKES 4 SERVINGS**

PREP TIME: 20 minutes
COOK TIME: 0 minutes

¼ cup Keto Mayonnaise
(page 225)

4 Almond Flour Tortillas
(page 20)

8 ounces sliced deli turkey

4 bacon slices, cooked

4 slices Monterey Jack cheese

1 small tomato, sliced thinly

2 or 3 lettuce leaves, chopped

PER SERVING: Calories: 508;
Total carbs: 13g; **Net carbs: 12g, 10%;**
Total fat: 36g, 64%; Protein: 33g, 26%;
Fiber: 1g; Sugar: 4g

VARIATION 1: Calories: 399;
Total carbs: 10g; **Net carbs: 9g, 10%;**
Total fat: 27g, 61%; Protein: 29g, 29%;
Fiber: 1g; Sugar: 2g

VARIATION 2: Calories: 281;
Total carbs: 9g; **Net carbs: 8g, 13%;**
Total fat: 21g, 67%; Protein: 14g, 20%;
Fiber: 1g; Sugar: 2g

Assemble the wraps: Spread 1 tablespoon of mayonnaise over each tortilla. Layer 2 ounces of sliced turkey, 1 bacon slice, 1 cheese slice, a few tomato slices, and some lettuce in the center of each. Wrap them up and slice each into 6 pieces. Serve immediately or refrigerate in an airtight container for up to 4 days.

VARIATION 1 **HAM AND CHEESE PINWHEELS:** Instead of mayo, use 1 tablespoon cream cheese per wrap. Layer 2 ounces ham and a slice of Swiss or Cheddar cheese in each tortilla. Follow the rest of the recipe as written.

VARIATION 2 **VEGGIE WRAPS:** Fill each wrap with 1 tablespoon cream cheese and a few ounces each julienned cucumber, spinach, and sliced radish. Season with salt and pepper, and wrap (no need to slice into pinwheels).

BACON CHEDDAR CAULIFLOWER SOUP

This is a keto take on cheesy potato soup using cauliflower instead of potatoes and adding a lot of delicious bacon. I like roasting the cauliflower first and adding it to a saucepan with some bacon fat to cook down before adding the heavy cream, Cheddar cheese, and a generous serving of crumbled bacon. This is homemade keto goodness at its finest—warm, filling, and super comforting, all in one bite. **MAKES 6 SERVINGS**

PREP TIME: 15 minutes
COOK TIME: 30 minutes

1 large head cauliflower, chopped into florets

¼ cup olive oil

Salt

Freshly ground black pepper

12 ounces bacon, chopped

½ onion, roughly chopped

2 garlic cloves, minced

2 cups chicken broth, or vegetable broth, plus more as needed

2 cups heavy (whipping) cream, plus more as needed

½ cup shredded Cheddar cheese, plus more for topping

Sliced scallion, green parts only, or fresh chives, for garnish

PER SERVING (about 1 cup):
Calories: 545; Total carbs: 11g;
**Net carbs: 7g, 8%; Total fat: 49g, 81%;
Protein: 15g, 11%;** Fiber: 4g; Sugar: 4g

VARIATION 1: Calories: 477;
Total carbs: 10g; **Net carbs: 6g, 9%;
Total fat: 41g, 77%; Protein: 17g, 14%;**
Fiber: 4g; Sugar: 4g

VARIATION 2: Calories: 546;
Total carbs: 11g; **Net carbs: 7g, 8%;
Total fat: 49g, 81%; Protein: 15g, 11%;**
Fiber: 4g; Sugar: 4g

1. Preheat the oven to 400°F.

2. On a large rimmed baking sheet, toss the cauliflower with the olive oil and season with salt and pepper. Bake for 25 to 30 minutes or until slightly browned.

3. While the cauliflower roasts, in a large saucepan over medium heat, cook the bacon for 5 to 7 minutes until crispy. Transfer the bacon to a paper towel-lined plate to drain; leave the bacon fat in the pan.

4. Return the pan to medium heat and add the onion and garlic. Stir well to combine and sauté for 5 to 7 minutes until the onion is softened and translucent. Season with salt and pepper.

5. Remove the cauliflower from the oven and add it to the pan with the onion and garlic. Stir in the broth and bring the liquid to a simmer. Reduce the heat to low. Cook for 5 to 7 minutes. Remove from the heat. With an immersion blender, carefully blend the soup. Alternatively, transfer the soup to a regular blender (working in batches if necessary), blend until smooth, and return the soup to the pan.

6. Stir in the cream. You may need to add a bit more broth or cream, depending on how thick you like your soup. Add the Cheddar and stir until melted and combined. Spoon the soup into bowls and top with bacon and more Cheddar. Garnish with scallion.

VARIATION 1 CAULIFLOWER CHEDDAR SOUP WITH PANCETTA: Substitute diced pancetta for the bacon. Follow the rest of the recipe as written.

VARIATION 2 SPICY BACON CHEDDAR CAULIFLOWER SOUP: Add 1 diced jalapeño pepper to the pan with the garlic and onion.

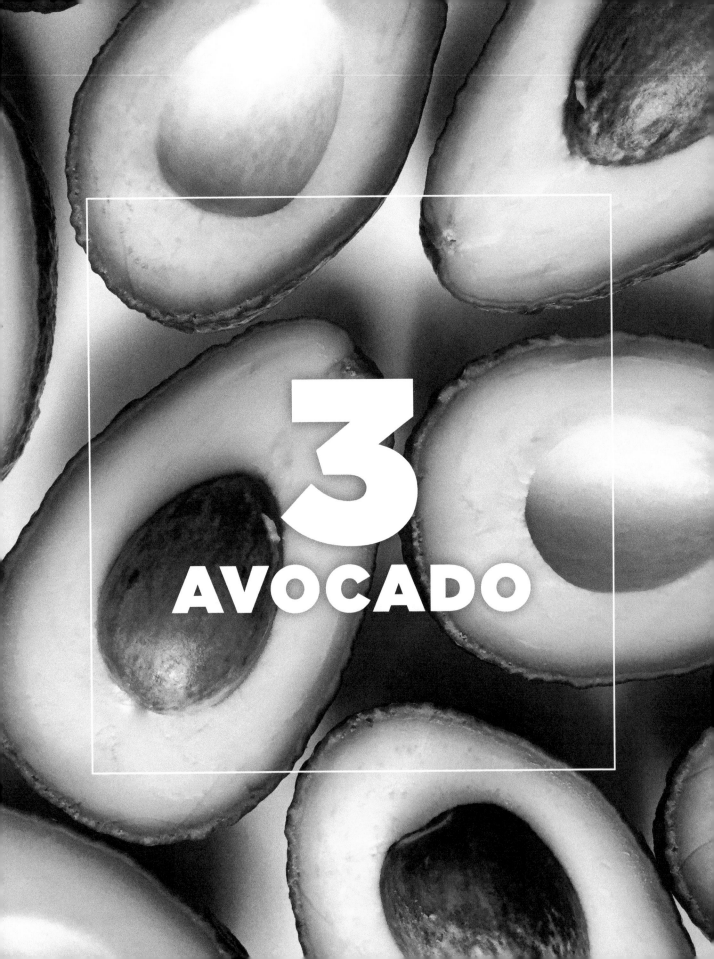

3
AVOCADO

I hope you like avocados, because on the keto diet they're about to become your new best friend. My husband and I serve at least a quarter of an avocado with just about everything—as a side with eggs, on top of a burger or salad, or on its own with a little salt and lime juice. Sometimes, at the end of the day, I am up to my limit for carbs and even protein, so avocado is a great way to up my fat intake without throwing off the balance of the rest of my macros.

It's kind of the perfect keto food—not very much protein, tons of fat, and enough dietary fiber that there are virtually no carbs. Also, it's delicious on, in, or beside pretty much anything; the flavor is so mild that it can be incorporated in a variety of dishes. In this chapter you'll find breakfast and lunch options, snacks, appetizers, and even some dessert ideas.

BAKED BREAKFAST AVOCADOS

These baked breakfast avocados are a variation of Paleo Omelet Muffins, a recipe from my first cookbook. Making the omelets in avocados cuts down on cleaning time (always a plus) and adds a lot of fat to the recipe (another plus when attempting to stay in ketosis). This basic recipe is easily customizable so you can include any meats or veggies you might need to use up.

MAKES 2 SERVINGS

PREP TIME: 10 minutes
COOK TIME: 20 minutes

1 ripe avocado, halved and pitted

4 eggs

2 ounces Canadian bacon, or other cooked ham, chopped

2 ounces shredded Cheddar cheese

Salt

Freshly ground black pepper

PER SERVING: Calories: 386; Total carbs: 10g; **Net carbs: 3g, 10%; Total fat: 30g, 70%; Protein: 19g, 20%;** Fiber: 7g; Sugar: 1g

VARIATION 1: Calories: 462; Total carbs: 11g; **Net carbs: 4g, 10%; Total fat: 38g, 74%; Protein: 19g, 16%;** Fiber: 7g; Sugar: 2g

VARIATION 2: Calories: 386; Total carbs: 10g; **Net carbs: 3g, 10%; Total fat: 30g, 70%; Protein: 19g, 20%;** Fiber: 7g; Sugar: 1g

1. Preheat the oven to 350°F.

2. Carefully scoop most of the avocado flesh into a medium bowl, leaving a layer of avocado intact with the peel.

3. Add the eggs to the avocado flesh and stir well to combine.

4. Stir in the Canadian bacon and season with salt and pepper. Spoon half the egg mixture into each avocado shell and top with the Cheddar. Bake for 20 to 30 minutes or until the eggs are set. Refrigerate leftovers in an airtight container for up to 3 days. To reheat, cover them with aluminum foil so they don't dry out and place them in a 350°F oven for 15 to 20 minutes.

VARIATION 1 **BAKED SAUSAGE BREAKFAST AVOCADOS:** Substitute chopped cooked breakfast sausage for the ham, and follow the rest of the recipe as written.

VARIATION 2 **BAKED (OVER-MEDIUM) BREAKFAST AVOCADOS:** Instead of blending the eggs with the other ingredients, mix together the scooped avocado and Canadian bacon and fill the halved avocados with it. Top each half with 2 cracked eggs and season with salt and pepper. Top with cheese and bake at 350°F for 15 to 20 minutes until the whites have set but the yolks are still runny.

MINT CHOCOLATE AVOCADO SMOOTHIE

After a while, keto and Paleo breakfasts can get boring. I know that every two to three weeks I get tired of eggs, so it's nice to have a couple smoothies on rotation to mix things up. Unfortunately, fruit smoothies don't fit well into a keto diet, but this mint chocolate avocado smoothie definitely does—and the good news is, it tastes like a milk shake. **MAKES 1 SMOOTHIE**

PREP TIME: 5 minutes
COOK TIME: 0 minutes

½ ripe avocado

1 cup heavy (whipping) cream, plus more as needed

1 to 2 tablespoons unsweetened cocoa powder

5 fresh mint leaves, or 1 teaspoon peppermint extract

½ cup ice

PER SERVING: Calories: 1105;
Total carbs: 22g; **Net carbs: 11g, 8%;**
Total fat: 109g, 89%; Protein: 9g, 3%;
Fiber: 11g; Sugar: 1g

VARIATION 1: Calories: 1117;
Total carbs: 25g; **Net carbs: 13g, 9%;**
Total fat: 109g, 88%; Protein: 9g, 3%;
Fiber: 12g; Sugar: 2g

VARIATION 2: Calories: 1117;
Total carbs: 23g; **Net carbs: 11g, 8%;**
Total fat: 109g, 88%; Protein: 11g, 6%;
Fiber: 12g; Sugar: 1g

In a blender, combine the avocado, cream, cocoa powder, mint, and ice. Blend until smooth. If necessary, add a bit more cream (or even a little water). Serve immediately.

VARIATION 1 **CHOCOLATE RASPBERRY AVOCADO SMOOTHIE:** If you have a little more room for carbs in your diet, skip the mint and add ¼ cup fresh or frozen raspberries to the smoothie.

VARIATION 2 **MINT CHOCOLATE AVOCADO SMOOTHIE WITH SPINACH:** Add some extra greens to your day by including 2 generous handfuls raw spinach to the mix.

ALLERGEN TIP: Swap out heavy cream for unsweetened almond milk or unsweetened coconut milk if you don't tolerate dairy.

EVERYDAY GUACAMOLE

I make guacamole regularly on the ketogenic diet, as a dip for veggies or as a topping or side with virtually any main dish. It's a delicious way to get a healthy serving of fat, and, once you give up the notion that guacamole belongs with tortilla chips, you'll realize it's great on its own as a snack! I like mine with lots of lime juice, which makes it super tasty and also helps it keep its nice bright green color—an added bonus. **MAKES 4 SERVINGS**

PREP TIME: 10 minutes
COOK TIME: 0 minutes

2 or 3 ripe avocados, peeled and pitted

¼ onion, minced

2 to 3 tablespoons salsa (I love Trader Joe's Salsa Autentica)

1 to 2 tablespoons chopped fresh cilantro (optional, but recommended)

Juice of 1 lime

½ teaspoon minced garlic

Salt

Freshly ground black pepper

1. In a large bowl or container (I make mine in a container with a lid so any leftovers are ready to go into the refrigerator), mash the avocados with a fork.

2. Add the onion, salsa, cilantro (if using), lime juice, and garlic. Season with salt and pepper and mix well until completely combined. Refrigerate leftovers in an airtight container for up to 3 days.

VARIATION 1 **EXTRA-SPICY GUACAMOLE:** Add 1 fresh jalapeño pepper (halved, seeded, and finely diced) to the guacamole ingredients.

VARIATION 2 **GREEK YOGURT GUACAMOLE:** Change the flavor profile slightly by adding ¼ to ½ cup Greek yogurt to the rest of the ingredients.

PER SERVING: Calories: 333;
Total carbs: 15g; **Net carbs: 4g, 18%;**
Total fat: 29g, 78%; Protein: 3g, 4%;
Fiber: 11g; Sugar: 2g

VARIATION 1: Calories: 334;
Total carbs: 16g; **Net carbs: 5g, 19%;**
Total fat: 29g, 78%; Protein: 3g, 3%;
Fiber: 11g; Sugar: 2g

VARIATION 2: Calories: 362;
Total carbs: 17g; **Net carbs: 6g, 19%;**
Total fat: 30g, 75%; Protein: 6g, 6%;
Fiber: 11g; Sugar: 3g

PERFECT PAIR: Serve this guacamole as a side with Turkey Club Pinwheels (page 32).

AVOCADO SALSA

This salsa is kind of like guacamole, only it's not all mashed together. It's a great complement to fish (Keto Fish Cakes with Garlic Aioli, page 126) or chicken (Easy Marinated Chicken Thighs, page 89). You can make it ahead of time and keep it in the refrigerator; just don't skimp on the lime juice or the avocados will turn brown. **MAKES 4 SERVINGS**

PREP TIME: 10 minutes
COOK TIME: 0 minutes

2 or 3 avocados, peeled, pitted, and diced

¼ red onion, diced

1 garlic clove, minced

Zest of ½ lime

Juice of 1 lime

¼ cup olive oil

Salt

Freshly ground black pepper

¼ cup chopped fresh cilantro

PER SERVING: Calories: 450;
Total carbs: 15g; **Net carbs: 5g, 13%;**
Total fat: 42g, 84%; Protein: 3g, 3%;
Fiber: 10g; Sugar: 1g

VARIATION 1: Calories: 450;
Total carbs: 15g; **Net carbs: 5g, 13%;**
Total fat: 42g, 84%; Protein: 3g, 3%;
Fiber: 10g; Sugar: 1g

VARIATION 2: Calories: 454;
Total carbs: 16g; **Net carbs: 5g, 13%;**
Total fat: 42g, 84%; Protein: 3g, 3%;
Fiber: 11g; Sugar: 1g

In a large bowl, gently toss together the diced avocados, onion, garlic, lime zest and juice, and olive oil. Season with salt and pepper. Cover and refrigerate in an airtight container for up to 4 days. Top with the cilantro before serving.

VARIATION 1 **SPICY AVOCADO SALSA:** Stir in ½ seeded and diced jalapeño pepper.

VARIATION 2 **AVOCADO SALSA WITH TOMATOES:** Toss in ½ cup halved grape tomatoes.

AVOCADO FRIES

These avocado fries are a tasty variation of my Bacon-Wrapped Avocados (page 41). They're breaded in almond flour and actually get a little crispy in the oven, which can be a welcome change when you're eating a keto diet. I love serving these as a side with almost anything from the second half of this book, especially Uncle Marty's Chicken (page 90) or The Classic Juicy Lucy (page 102). **MAKES 2 SERVINGS**

PREP TIME: 10 minutes
COOK TIME: 20 minutes

Nonstick olive oil cooking spray, or olive oil

1 cup almond flour

¼ teaspoon garlic powder

¼ teaspoon onion powder

Salt

Freshly ground black pepper

1 egg

2 large avocados, halved and pitted, each half cut into 4 or 5 slices

PER SERVING: Calories: 436; Total carbs: 19g; **Net carbs: 6g, 17%; Total fat: 36g, 74%; Protein: 9g, 9%;** Fiber: 13g; Sugar: 1g

VARIATION 1: Calories: 490; Total carbs: 19g; **Net carbs: 6g, 16%; Total fat: 42g, 77%; Protein: 9g, 8%;** Fiber: 13g; Sugar: 1g

VARIATION 2: Calories: 723; Total carbs: 19g; **Net carbs: 5g, 11%; Total fat: 67g, 83%; Protein: 11g, 6%;** Fiber: 14g; Sugar: 1g

1. Preheat the oven to 425°F.

2. Spray a baking sheet with olive oil spray or coat with a little olive oil.

3. Place the almond flour in a shallow dish and season it with the garlic powder, onion powder, and some salt and pepper.

4. In another shallow dish, whisk the egg.

5. Dip both sides of each avocado slice first into the egg and then into the seasoned almond flour. Cover both sides with the flour and place on the prepared baking sheet. Spray the fries with a fine mist of cooking spray.

6. Bake for 15 to 20 minutes or until the almond flour browns slightly. Remove from the oven and serve immediately.

VARIATION 1 **PAN-FRIED AVOCADO FRIES:** Brown the avocado fries in a skillet instead of the oven: use about 1 tablespoon olive oil and cook over medium-high heat for 2 to 3 minutes per side.

VARIATION 2 **AVOCADO FRIES WITH CHIPOTLE AIOLI:** In a blender, mix ½ cup Keto Mayonnaise (page 225) with 2 canned chiles in adobo sauce. Season with salt and pepper and serve as a dipping sauce for the avocado fries.

PERFECT PAIR: Serve these with Bacon Cheddar Ranch Dip (page 24).

BACON-WRAPPED AVOCADOS

This recipe is a go-to whenever we have people over or I want to impress someone with hors d'oeuvres before dinner but don't have a ton of time. The best part is that I always have avocados and bacon on hand, so I can make these with little to no notice. They make a fantastic appetizer and all you need is a skillet and about 20 minutes to make it happen! **MAKES 4 SERVINGS**

PREP TIME: 10 minutes
COOK TIME: 15 minutes

8 bacon slices

1 ripe avocado, peeled and cut into 8 wedges

Salt

Freshly ground black pepper

1 or 2 lime wedges

Ground cayenne pepper

PER SERVING: Calories: 314; Total carbs: 5g; **Net carbs: 2g, 6%; Total fat: 26g, 75%; Protein: 15g, 19%;** Fiber: 3g; Sugar: 0g

VARIATION 1: Calories: 165; Total carbs: 4g; **Net carbs: 1g, 10%; Total fat: 13g, 71%; Protein: 8g, 19%;** Fiber:3 g; Sugar: 0g

VARIATION 2: Calories: 314; Total carbs: 5g; **Net carbs: 2g, 6%; Total fat: 26g, 75%; Protein: 15g, 19%;** Fiber: 3g; Sugar: 0g

1. Wrap 1 bacon slice around each avocado wedge. If needed, use a toothpick to secure them.

2. Heat a nonstick skillet over medium-high heat. Evenly space the bacon-wrapped wedges around the skillet. If you aren't using a toothpick, place the loose end of the bacon facing down to create a seal as it cooks. Cook for 6 to 8 minutes, turning every couple of minutes until the bacon is cooked.

3. Remove from the heat and finish with a sprinkle of salt, pepper, lime juice, and cayenne. Serve warm.

VARIATION 1 **PROSCIUTTO-WRAPPED AVOCADOS:** Instead of bacon, use 1 slice prosciutto to wrap each avocado wedge. Omit the lime juice and cayenne and season only with salt and pepper, if desired.

VARIATION 2 **BACON-WRAPPED AVOCADOS IN THE OVEN:** Place all the bacon-wrapped avocado wedges on a baking sheet and bake at 350°F for 15 to 20 minutes or until the bacon is cooked through. This saves a lot of time if you're making a large number and don't want to do them in batches on the stove top.

INGREDIENT TIP: Use precooked bacon instead of raw bacon if you're short on time. You can heat them quickly in a skillet, or even in the microwave, for about 1 minute.

CHICKEN SALAD-STUFFED AVOCADOS

This is one of my favorite easy lunches; you can make the chicken salad ahead of time and spoon it into avocados for a nice bit of extra fat. I always keep avocados on hand but sometimes get a little sick of eating them on their own as a side with everything, so this is a fun way to incorporate the avocado into the dish itself. **MAKES 4 SERVINGS**

PREP TIME: 10 minutes
COOK TIME: 0 minutes

2 large avocados, halved and pitted

1 (12.5-ounce) can chicken, drained

½ cup Keto Mayonnaise (page 225)

½ celery stalk, diced

1 or 2 scallions, green parts only, thinly sliced

Salt

Freshly ground black pepper

1. Scoop about 2 tablespoons of avocado flesh from each half into a medium bowl.

2. Add the chicken, mayonnaise, celery, and scallions. Season with salt and pepper and stir together until combined.

3. Spoon the chicken salad into the avocado halves and serve. Refrigerate leftovers in an airtight container for up to 3 days.

VARIATION 1 **TUNA SALAD-STUFFED AVOCADOS:** Use tuna instead of chicken and add the juice of ½ lemon.

VARIATION 2 **EGG SALAD-STUFFED AVOCADOS:** Stuff the avocado halves with Egg Salad (page 11) instead of chicken salad.

MAKE AHEAD: Make the chicken salad up to 5 days ahead, and stuff the avocado halves right before serving.

PER SERVING: Calories: 585;
Total carbs: 9g; **Net carbs: 2g, 7%;**
Total fat: 49g, 75%; Protein: 27g, 18%;
Fiber: 7g; Sugar: 1g

VARIATION 1: Calories: 520;
Total carbs: 9g; **Net carbs: 2g, 6%;**
Total fat: 44g, 76%; Protein: 23g, 18%;
Fiber: 7g; Sugar: 1g

VARIATION 2: Calories: 488;
Total carbs: 10g; **Net carbs: 3g, 8%;**
Total fat:44 g, 81%; Protein: 13g, 11%;
Fiber: 7g; Sugar: 1g

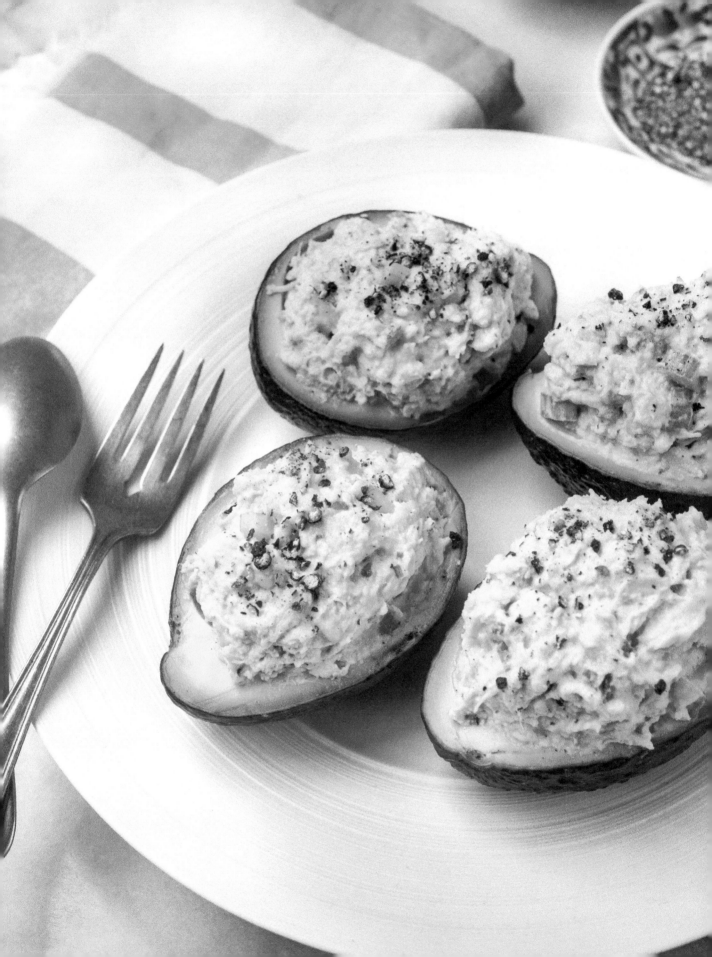

SHRIMP LOUIE AVOCADO STACKERS

This is a very simplified version of a shrimp (or crab) Louie salad. Basically I've just kept my favorite parts: the seafood, the avocado, and the dressing. This makes a nice quick lunch or snack, or even an appetizer that's sure to please. The chilled juicy shrimp, creamy avocado, and tangy Louie dressing are a winning combination. **MAKES 2 SERVINGS**

PREP TIME: 15 minutes
COOK TIME: 0 minutes

¼ cup Keto Mayonnaise (page 225)

1 tablespoon Low-Carb Ketchup (page 226)

Hot sauce

⅛ teaspoon smoked paprika

⅛ teaspoon chili powder

Salt

Freshly ground black pepper

6 ounces cooked shrimp, roughly chopped

1 large avocado, peeled, halved, and pitted, halves cut lengthwise into thick slices

2 lemon wedges

PER SERVING: Calories: 435;
Total carbs: 17g; **Net carbs: 10g, 16%;**
Total fat: 31g, 64%; Protein: 22g, 20%;
Fiber: 7g; Sugar: 2g

VARIATION 1: Calories: 419;
Total carbs: 16g; **Net carbs: 9g, 15%;**
Total fat: 31g, 67%; Protein: 19g, 18%;
Fiber: 7g; Sugar: 2g

VARIATION 2: Calories: 511;
Total carbs: 21g; **Net carbs: 13g, 16%;**
Total fat: 35g, 62%; Protein: 28g, 22%;
Fiber: 8g; Sugar: 5g

1. In a large bowl, whisk together the mayonnaise, ketchup, a few dashes of hot sauce, paprika, and chili powder. Season with salt and pepper.

2. Add the shrimp, stirring to thoroughly combine the dressing and shrimp.

3. Layer a few avocado slices on each of two plates. Spoon the shrimp on top. Serve immediately with a lemon wedge.

VARIATION 1 **CRAB LOUIE AVOCADO STACKERS:** Substitute cooked crabmeat for the shrimp. Follow the rest of the recipe as written.

VARIATION 2 **TRADITIONAL LOUIE SALAD:** Instead of this abbreviated version, enjoy a full shrimp Louie salad: For each salad arrange ½ small head butter lettuce, sliced avocado, ½ Roma tomato, 1 halved hardboiled egg, and a few slices of cucumber and radish. Serve with a side of Louie dressing.

AVOCADO SALAD WITH ARUGULA AND RED ONION

I'm a huge fan of arugula; for some reason, its peppery bite reminds me of my grandfather Albino, whom I never met. He was a great cook and had an awesome garden full of vegetables; as a kid I must have heard stories of how he loved arugula and held onto it, almost like my own memory of him. This avocado salad with arugula and red onion is delicious and easy; I think he would have liked it. **MAKES 2 SERVINGS**

PREP TIME: 10 minutes
COOK TIME: 0 minutes

   DF **GF** **NF**

2 cups arugula, washed and dried

¼ red onion, thinly sliced

½ cup olive oil

¼ cup balsamic vinegar

1 tablespoon Dijon mustard

Salt

Freshly ground black pepper

1 avocado, peeled, halved, pitted, and diced or sliced

PER SERVING: Calories: 686; Total carbs: 11g; **Net carbs: 3g, 6%;** **Total fat: 70g, 92%; Protein: 3g, 2%;** Fiber: 8g; Sugar: 2g

VARIATION 1: Calories: 904; Total carbs: 11g; **Net carbs: 3g, 5%;** **Total fat: 76g, 76%; Protein: 44g, 19%;** Fiber: 8g; Sugar: 2g

VARIATION 2: Calories: 1134; Total carbs: 12g; **Net carbs: 4g, 5%;** **Total fat: 90g, 71%; Protein: 69g, 24%;** Fiber: 8g; Sugar: 2g

1. In a large bowl, combine the arugula and red onion.

2. In a small bowl, whisk together the olive oil, vinegar, mustard, and some salt and pepper. Pour the dressing over the salad and toss well to combine.

3. Divide the salad between two bowls and top each with half an avocado. Season with a bit more salt and pepper and serve.

VARIATION 1 **STEAK AND AVOCADO SALAD WITH ARUGULA AND RED ONION:** Add 3 to 4 ounces grilled steak to each salad, such as my Grilled Soy Lime Flank Steak (page 105).

VARIATION 2 **BAKED SALMON AND AVOCADO SALAD WITH ARUGULA AND RED ONION:** Top each salad with a serving of Oven-Baked Dijon Salmon (page 134).

CHILLED CILANTRO AND AVOCADO SOUP

When it's just too hot to cook, a chilled soup can be the perfect meal. I wasn't really into chilled soups until my husband and I moved to the Bay Area, which, in the summer, is much cooler than North Carolina, Virginia, and Minnesota. We don't have central air because of that, so when it is hot, we really feel it. This creamy but spicy avocado soup is perfect for those hot afternoons when you just don't have it in you to stand over the stove. **MAKES 6 SERVINGS**

PREP TIME: 10 minutes
COOK TIME: 7 minutes
CHILLING TIME: 3 hours

2 to 3 tablespoons olive oil

1 large white onion, diced

3 garlic cloves, crushed

1 serrano chile, seeded and diced

Salt

Freshly ground black pepper

4 or 5 ripe avocados, peeled, halved, and pitted

4 cups chicken broth, or vegetable broth

2 cups water

Juice of 1 lemon

¼ cup chopped fresh cilantro, plus more for garnish

½ cup sour cream

PER SERVING: Calories: 513; Total carbs: 20g; **Net carbs: 8g, 16%; Total fat: 45g, 79%; Protein: 7g, 5%;** Fiber: 12g; Sugar: 2g

VARIATION 1: Calories: 647; Total carbs: 21g; **Net carbs: 9g, 13%; Total fat: 59g, 82%; Protein: 8g, 5%;** Fiber:12 g; Sugar: 3g

VARIATION 2: Calories: 517; Total carbs: 20g; **Net carbs: 8g, 16%; Total fat: 45g, 79%; Protein: 7g, 5%;** Fiber: 12g; Sugar: 2g

1. In a large pan over medium heat, heat the olive oil.

2. Add the onion and garlic. Sauté for 5 to 7 minutes until the onion is softened and translucent.

3. Add the serrano, season with salt and pepper, and remove from the heat.

4. In a blender, combine the avocados, chicken broth, water, lemon juice, cilantro, and onion-garlic-chile mixture. Purée until smooth (you may have to do this in batches), strain through a fine-mesh sieve, and season with more salt and pepper. Refrigerate, covered, for about 3 hours or until chilled through.

5. To serve, top with sour cream and a sprinkle of chopped cilantro. Refrigerate leftovers in an airtight container for up to 1 week.

VARIATION 1 **CREAMY CHILLED CILANTRO AND AVOCADO SOUP:** Substitute heavy (whipping) cream for the water to get even more fat and lusciousness into this soup.

VARIATION 2 **CHILLED CILANTRO AND AVOCADO SOUP WITH CUCUMBER:** Add ½ large peeled cucumber to the blender with the other ingredients. Serve the soup with the remaining half cucumber diced on top.

MAKE AHEAD: You can make this ahead of time and chill overnight before serving.

CHOCOLATE AVOCADO PUDDING

I make this pudding whenever I'm in the mood for a treat but don't want too much sugar. Sometimes low-carb desserts can be hard to make or involve a lot of ingredients, but this one is practically effortless and comes together in fewer than 10 minutes. I always have avocados on hand, and my pantry is always stocked with unsweetened cocoa powder, so I'm always ready to make this pudding! **MAKES 4 SERVINGS**

PREP TIME: 10 minutes
COOK TIME: 0 minutes

2 ripe avocados, peeled, halved, and pitted

⅓ cup plus ¼ cup unsweetened cocoa powder

½ teaspoon vanilla extract

1 teaspoon liquid stevia

Pinch salt

PER SERVING: Calories: 264; Total carbs: 16g; **Net carbs: 5g, 24%;** **Total fat: 20g, 68%; Protein: 5g, 8%;** Fiber: 11g; Sugar: 1g

VARIATION 1: Calories: 313; Total carbs: 17g; **Net carbs: 5g, 22%;** **Total fat: 25g, 72%; Protein: 5g, 6%;** Fiber: 12g; Sugar: 1g

VARIATION 2: Calories: 286; Total carbs: 17g; **Net carbs: 5g, 24%;** **Total fat: 22g, 69%; Protein: 5g, 7%;** Fiber: 12g; Sugar: 1g

In a food processor, combine the avocados, cocoa powder, vanilla, stevia, and salt. Blend until smooth. Transfer to a piping bag (or a plastic bag with the tip cut off) and pipe into individual dishes. Serve immediately, or cover and refrigerate for up to 1 week.

VARIATION 1 **CINNAMON MACADAMIA CHOCOLATE AVOCADO PUDDING:** Add 1 teaspoon ground cinnamon to the pudding and top each serving with 1 tablespoon crushed macadamia nuts.

VARIATION 2 **CHOCOLATE AVOCADO PUDDING WITH HAZELNUTS:** Top each serving with 1 tablespoon crushed hazelnuts.

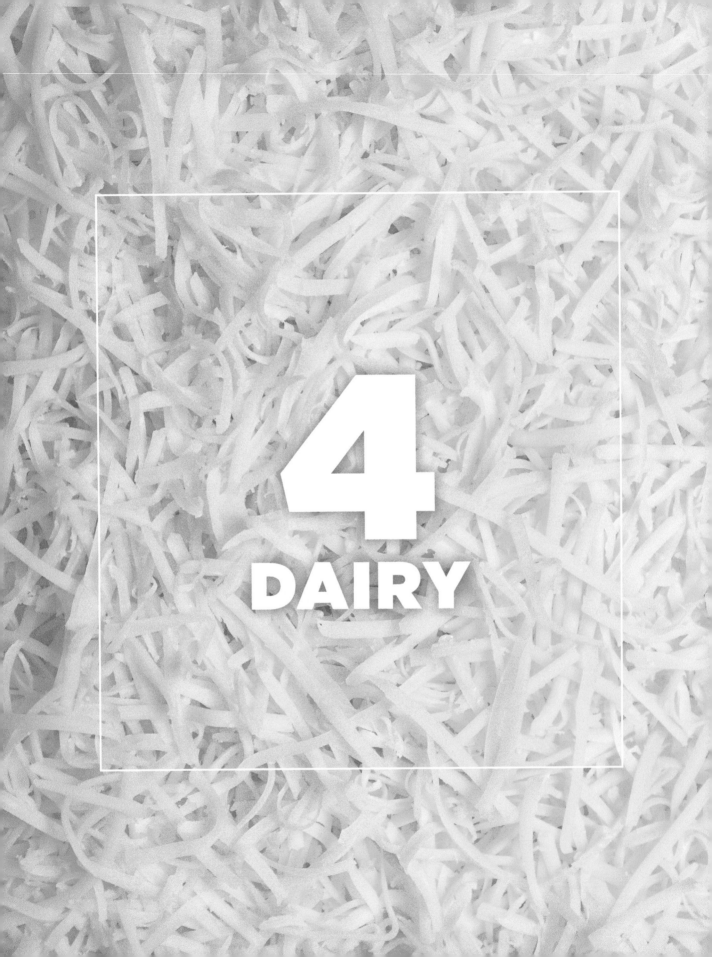

4
DAIRY

I decided to name this chapter "Dairy" instead of focusing on one ingredient such as cream cheese or Greek yogurt, because there are several dairy products that fit very well into the keto diet. However, it needs to be said that not all dairy works—*always avoid anything low fat or nonfat and always choose the product with the highest fat content*—even 2% and whole milk have more carbs than necessary, so when it comes to milk, stick to heavy cream or half-and-half.

The dairy products I use most are cream cheese, Cheddar cheese (I think it goes with everything and also makes an easy snack), and heavy cream (either in cooking or in my coffee or tea). The following recipes range from breakfasts to quick lunches and lots of snacks. I don't consider dairy to be a huge keto staple, but it's hard to make the diet work without it. (If you're dairy-free, check out some of the recipe tips for dairy-free alternatives, or skip this chapter and focus more on the avocado and nut chapters—those are good ingredients to ensure you're incorporating enough fat into your diet.)

GREEK YOGURT PEANUT BUTTER SMOOTHIE

My friend Paige makes the most amazing peanut butter dip—we just call it "peanut butter dip"—and we have it pretty much every time we hang out together (funny side note: my dog loves it, too). Anyway, this smoothie is a keto version of that dip, in breakfast form. **MAKES 1 SMOOTHIE**

PREP TIME: 5 minutes
COOK TIME: 0 minutes

¼ cup unsweetened peanut butter

½ cup plain Greek yogurt

½ cup water, plus more as needed

½ cup heavy (whipping) cream, plus more as needed

1 tablespoon unsweetened cocoa powder

Ice

PER SERVING: Calories: 692; Total carbs: 21g; **Net carbs: 15g, 12%; Total fat: 56g, 73%; Protein: 26g, 15%;** Fiber: 6g; Sugar: 8g

VARIATION 1: Calories: 814 ; Total carbs: 25g; **Net carbs: 19g, 12%; Total fat: 58g, 62%; Protein: 48g, 30%;** Fiber: 6g; Sugar: 9g

VARIATION 2: Calories: 818; Total carbs: 21g; **Net carbs: 15g, 10%; Total fat: 70g, 77%; Protein: 26g, 13%;** Fiber: 6g; Sugar: 8g

In a blender, combine the peanut butter, yogurt, water, heavy cream, cocoa powder, and a small handful of ice cubes. Blend until smooth. If it's too thick, add another splash of water or cream. Serve immediately.

VARIATION 1 **PROTEIN POWDER GREEK YOGURT AND PEANUT BUTTER SMOOTHIE:** If you have a keto-friendly protein powder you like, skip the chocolate and add a scoop of that to the smoothie.

VARIATION 2 **GREEK YOGURT PEANUT BUTTER SMOOTHIE WITH COCONUT OIL:** Add some extra fat to this smoothie with 1 tablespoon coconut oil.

ALLERGEN TIP: Use canned coconut cream instead of heavy cream if you don't tolerate dairy.

KETO PANCAKES

These keto pancakes are a lifesaver during the first month of low-carb eating when you generally get a little bored with scrambled eggs (or eggs any style, for that matter). I still love this recipe because of its ease: you throw all the ingredients into a blender then just pour it into the skillet. With just a few ingredients, these pancakes are super simple, super decadent, and totally fit into a ketogenic diet! **MAKES 2 SERVINGS**

PREP TIME: 5 minutes
COOK TIME: 10 minutes

4 eggs

4 ounces cream cheese

¼ cup almond flour

⅔ teaspoon baking powder

⅔ teaspoon ground cinnamon, plus more for sprinkling (optional)

1 teaspoon vanilla extract

1 tablespoon butter, plus more for serving

PER SERVING: Calories: 404; Total carbs: 4g; **Net carbs: 4g, 4%; Total fat: 36g, 80%; Protein: 16g, 16%;** Fiber: 0g; Sugar: 1g

VARIATION 1: Calories: 470; Total carbs: 6g; **Net carbs: 5g, 6%; Total fat: 42g, 80%; Protein: 17g, 14%;** Fiber: 1g; Sugar: 2g

VARIATION 2: Calories: 492; Total carbs: 5g; **Net carbs: 4g, 4%; Total fat: 40g, 73%; Protein: 28g, 23%;** Fiber: 1g; Sugar: 1g

1. In a blender, combine the eggs, cream cheese, almond flour, baking powder, cinnamon, and vanilla. Blend for about 2 minutes or until all the ingredients are completely combined. Give the blender a shake or tap it on the counter to get rid of any air bubbles in the batter.

2. Heat a large nonstick skillet over medium-high heat. Add some of the butter and stir to coat the bottom and edges of the pan. Pour a small amount of batter into the pan and cook for about 2 minutes until set. (I usually cook two at a time to prevent the pancakes from sticking together or flipping them onto each other.)

3. Flip the pancake(s) and cook for 2 to 3 minutes on the other side. Transfer to a plate.

4. Repeat with the remaining butter and batter. Serve the pancakes immediately with more butter and a sprinkle of cinnamon (if using).

VARIATION 1 **KETO PANCAKES WITH RASPBERRIES AND WHIPPED CREAM:** Serve this recipe with ¼ cup fresh raspberries (chopped or whole, it's up to you) and some whipped cream—beat heavy whipping cream until thick. Add a few drops (or a packet) of stevia (or other low-carb sweetener) to the whipped cream, if desired.

VARIATION 2 **HAM AND CHEESE KETO CRÊPES:** Because these pancakes are similar in texture to crêpes, skip the vanilla and cinnamon and serve them with sliced ham and cheese. Roll them up or fold them into triangles and enjoy hot.

MARINATED CHEESE

This marinated cheese is kind of famous in my family—my mom made it any-time we had people over, and my best friend and next-door neighbor, Patrick, loved it so much that his mom started making it, too. So, now, whenever our families gather together, you can bet there'll be marinated cheese. It's an awesome appetizer, but I also like making a batch and keeping it for a quick snack. It's really filling so you only need a few pieces at a time (but you'll want more). **MAKES 8 SERVINGS**

PREP TIME: 10 minutes
COOK TIME: 0 minutes
CHILLING TIME: 8 hours

½ cup olive oil

½ cup white wine vinegar

2 or 3 garlic cloves, minced

4 scallions, green parts only, thinly sliced

3 tablespoons chopped fresh parsley leaves

1 (2-ounce jar) diced pimientos, drained

Salt

Freshly ground black pepper

1 (8-ounce) block sharp Cheddar cheese, halved lengthwise and cut widthwise into ½-inch squares

1 (8-ounce) block cream cheese halved lengthwise and cut widthwise into ½-inch squares

1. In a small bowl, whisk together the olive oil, vinegar, garlic, scallions, parsley, pimientos, and season with some salt and pepper.

2. In a container with a lid, assemble the cheese (we like to alternate pieces of Cheddar and cream cheese for a prettier presentation) and cover with the marinade. Cover and refrigerate for at least 8 hours.

3. Remove from the refrigerator 15 to 20 minutes before serving, and transfer the cheese to a serving platter, pouring the marinade over the top. Refrigerate leftovers in an airtight container for up to 1 week.

PER SERVING: Calories: 336;
Total carbs: 2g; **Net carbs: 1g, 2%;**
Total fat: 32g, 86%; Protein: 10g, 12%;
Fiber: 0g; Sugar: 1g

VARIATION 1: Calories: 323;
Total carbs: 2g; **Net carbs: 1g, 3%;**
Total fat: 31g, 86%; Protein: 9g, 11%;
Fiber: 0g; Sugar: 1g

VARIATION 2: Calories: 336;
Total carbs: 2g; **Net carbs: 1g, 2%;**
Total fat: 32g, 86%; Protein: 10g, 12%;
Fiber: 0g; Sugar: 1g

VARIATION 1 **MARINATED CHEESE WITH MONTEREY JACK:**
Switch the Cheddar for Monterey Jack or any other kind of
cheese you like.

VARIATION 2 **SPICY MARINATED CHEESE:** Add ½ seeded and
diced jalapeño pepper to the marinade. Top with fresh chopped
cilantro.

CLASSIC QUESO DIP

I know, the first thing that comes to mind when you think of queso dip is tortilla chips—and margaritas—but I promise this dip is just as good with sliced veggies or drizzled over any of your favorite simply grilled proteins. I love it on chicken as a Mexican-inspired cheesy chicken dinner. Most queso dips use cheese products like Velveeta, but this one uses regular shredded cheese, which I usually prefer. **MAKES 4 SERVINGS**

PREP TIME: 5 minutes
COOK TIME: 10 to 15 minutes

3 tablespoons butter

¼ white onion, diced

1 jalapeño pepper, seeded and diced

½ cup heavy (whipping) cream

½ cup shredded Monterey Jack cheese

¼ cup shredded American cheese

2 to 3 tablespoons salsa

Salt

Freshly ground black pepper

1 to 2 tablespoons water (optional)

PER SERVING: Calories: 216; Total carbs: 3g; **Net carbs: 3g, 6%;** **Total fat: 20g, 83%; Protein: 6g, 11%;** Fiber: 0g; Sugar: 1g

VARIATION 1: Calories: 216; Total carbs: 3g; **Net carbs: 3g, 6%;** **Total fat: 20g, 83%; Protein: 6g, 11%;** Fiber: 0g; Sugar: 1g

VARIATION 2: Calories: 377; Total carbs: 4g; **Net carbs: 4g, 4%;** **Total fat: 33g, 79%; Protein: 16g, 17%;** Fiber: 0g; Sugar: 2g

1. In a small saucepan over medium heat, melt the butter.

2. Add the onion and jalapeño. Sauté for 5 to 7 minutes until the onion is softened and translucent.

3. Stir in the cream and bring to a gentle boil.

4. Add the Jack and American cheeses, a little at a time, and reduce the heat to low.

5. Add the salsa and stir well to combine it with the cheeses as they melt. Season with salt and pepper. If necessary, add a little water to thin the dip. Serve immediately. Refrigerate leftovers in an airtight container for up to 4 days.

VARIATION 1 **QUESO DIP WITH PEPPER JACK:** Add a little more heat to this dip with pepper jack instead of Monterey Jack.

VARIATION 2 **SPICY SAUSAGE CHEESE DIP:** Brown ½ pound spicy ground sausage in the saucepan with the onion and jalapeño. Add the remaining ingredients and follow the rest of the recipe as written.

EVERYTHING BAGEL CREAM CHEESE DIP

I love bagels—a lot. When I was in high school our literary magazine sold bagels every Thursday at break, and I invariably got an everything bagel with cream cheese and a slice of tomato (an order I stole from an English teacher I particularly admired). This dip combines all that garlic and salt and sesame goodness and is perfect for spreading on Almond Sesame Crackers (page 68) or just for dipping veggies into. I won't tell anyone if you eat it by itself.

MAKES 4 SERVINGS

PREP TIME: 10 minutes
COOK TIME: 0 minutes

1 (8-ounce) package cream cheese, at room temperature

½ cup sour cream

1 tablespoon garlic powder

1 tablespoon dried onion, or onion powder

1 tablespoon sesame seeds

1 tablespoon kosher salt

PER SERVING: Calories: 291; Total carbs: 6g; **Net carbs: 5g, 8%; Total fat: 27g, 84%; Protein: 6g, 8%;** Fiber: 1g; Sugar: 1g

VARIATION 1: Calories: 569; Total carbs: 15g; **Net carbs: 14g, 11%; Total fat: 45g, 71%; Protein: 26g, 18%;** Fiber: 1g; Sugar: 4g

VARIATION 2: Calories: 294; Total carbs: 7g; **Net carbs: 6g, 8%; Total fat: 27g, 84%; Protein: 6g, 8%;** Fiber: 1g; Sugar: 1g

In a small bowl, combine the cream cheese, sour cream, garlic powder, dried onion, sesame seeds, and salt. Stir well to incorporate everything together. Serve immediately or cover and refrigerate for up to 6 days.

VARIATION 1 **EVERYTHING BAGEL CREAM CHEESE DIP KETO ROLL-UPS:** Spread 1 tablespoon of this dip on Almond Flour Tortillas (page 20) and top with sliced tomatoes and turkey or ham. Roll up and serve immediately.

VARIATION 2 **EVERYTHING BAGEL CREAM CHEESE DIP WITH TOMATO:** Top this dip with 1 Roma tomato, diced.

KETO TZATZIKI SAUCE

The best thing about most dairy-based dips is that they're keto-friendly; this one is no different, especially finished with a nice drizzle of olive oil! The cucumber and fresh mint are a delicious combination and make a great side for dipping with some grilled chicken or beef. **MAKES 6 SERVINGS**

PREP TIME: 10 minutes
COOK TIME: 0 minutes

1 cup Greek yogurt

2 garlic cloves, minced

1 tablespoon olive oil

½ large cucumber (or 2 small), finely chopped

2 tablespoons fresh mint leaves, minced

Salt

Freshly ground black pepper

PER SERVING (¼ cup): Calories: 62; Total carbs: 4g; **Net carbs: 4g, 26%; Total fat: 2g, 30%; Protein: 7g, 44%;** Fiber: 0g; Sugar: 3g

VARIATION 1: Calories: 86; Total carbs: 4g; **Net carbs: 4g, 18%; Total fat: 6g, 64%; Protein: 4g, 18%;** Fiber: 0g; Sugar: 2g

VARIATION 2: Calories: 64; Total carbs: 4g; **Net carbs: 4g, 26%; Total fat: 2g, 30%; Protein: 7g, 44%;** Fiber: 0g; Sugar: 3g

In a large bowl, stir together the yogurt, garlic, olive oil, and cucumber. Add the mint and continue to stir. Season with salt and pepper. Serve immediately or keep refrigerated in an airtight container for up to 1 week.

VARIATION 1 **SOUR CREAM TZATZIKI:** Use half yogurt and half sour cream to increase the amount of fat in this dip.

VARIATION 2 **LEMON DILL TZATZIKI:** Add 2 tablespoons chopped fresh dill and the juice of ½ lemon to add even more flavor.

MAKE IT PALEO: Use Keto Mayonnaise (page 225) instead of yogurt to make this dip dairy-free and Paleo.

CHEESE CRISPS

These cheese crisps, similar to crackers, make a great keto snack when you're in the mood for something crunchy. All you need is cheese and an oven, which makes me like this recipe even more! I'm always so surprised by how many great keto recipes only call for a few ingredients but still result in flavorful, delicious food. **MAKES ABOUT 8 CRISPS**

PREP TIME: 5 minutes
COOK TIME: 15 minutes

½ cup shredded Mexican blend cheese

PER SERVING (1 crisp): Calories: 35; Total carbs: 0g; **Net carbs: 0g, 0%; Total fat: 3g, 77%; Protein: 2g, 23%;** Fiber: 0g; Sugar: 0g

VARIATION 1: Calories: 30; Total carbs: 1g; **Net carbs: 1g, 13%; Total fat: 2g, 60%; Protein: 2g, 27%;** Fiber: 0g; Sugar: 0g

VARIATION 2: Calories: 35; Total carbs: 0g; **Net carbs: 0g, 0%; Total fat: 3g, 77%; Protein: 2g, 23%;** Fiber: 0g; Sugar: 0g

1. Preheat the oven to 350°F.

2. Line a baking sheet with parchment paper or a silicone mat and arrange small piles of cheese (about 1 tablespoon each) about 2 inches apart. Pat them down so all the piles are equally thick. Bake for 13 to 15 minutes or until the cheese spreads slightly and begins to brown. Remove and cool completely before serving.

3. Refrigerate leftovers in an airtight container for up to 1 week.

VARIATION 1 **GARLIC PARMESAN CRISPS:** Use Parmesan instead of the Mexican blend for a variation in flavor. Sprinkle with 2 teaspoons garlic powder after baking.

VARIATION 2 **HERBED CHEESE CRISPS:** Sprinkle with 2 teaspoons herbes de Provence or your favorite dried herb/spice mix after baking.

KETO JALAPEÑO POPPERS

I used to make these jalapeño poppers with goat cheese, but lately I've been enjoying them even more with cream cheese, which I think complements the heat of the pepper more than goat cheese does, although both variations are delicious. You might be asking yourself what makes a jalapeño popper keto-friendly, and the answer, of course, is bacon! Instead of battering and frying these, they are wrapped in bacon and popped in the oven to broil.

MAKES 12 POPPERS

PREP TIME: 15 minutes
COOK TIME: 25 minutes

 GF NF

6 large jalapeño peppers, halved and seeded

4 ounces cream cheese, at room temperature

6 bacon slices, halved widthwise

PER SERVING (3 poppers):
Calories: 294; Total carbs: 3g;
**Net carbs: 2g, 3%; Total fat: 29g, 87%;
Protein: 7g, 10%;** Fiber: 1g; Sugar: 2g

VARIATION 1: Calories: 274;
Total carbs: 2g; **Net carbs: 1g, 2%;
Total fat: 25g, 82%; Protein: 10g, 16%;**
Fiber: 1g; Sugar: 1g

VARIATION 2: Calories: 386;
Total carbs:9 g; **Net carbs: 4g, 8%;
Total fat: 36g, 83%; Protein: 9g, 9%;**
Fiber: 5g; Sugar: 4g

1. Preheat the oven to 425°F.

2. Spoon cream cheese into each jalapeño half. Wrap each piece with a half bacon slice. Place on a rimmed baking sheet and bake for about 20 minutes until the bacon is cooked through but not yet completely crispy.

3. Turn the oven to broil, and broil the poppers for about 3 minutes to get them extra crispy. Cool slightly and serve warm.

VARIATION 1 **GOAT CHEESE JALAPEÑO POPPERS:** Instead of cream cheese, use goat cheese. Follow the rest of the recipe as written.

VARIATION 2 **AVOCADO-STUFFED JALAPEÑO POPPERS:** Add 1 slice of avocado to each popper before adding the cream cheese. Follow the rest of the recipe as written.

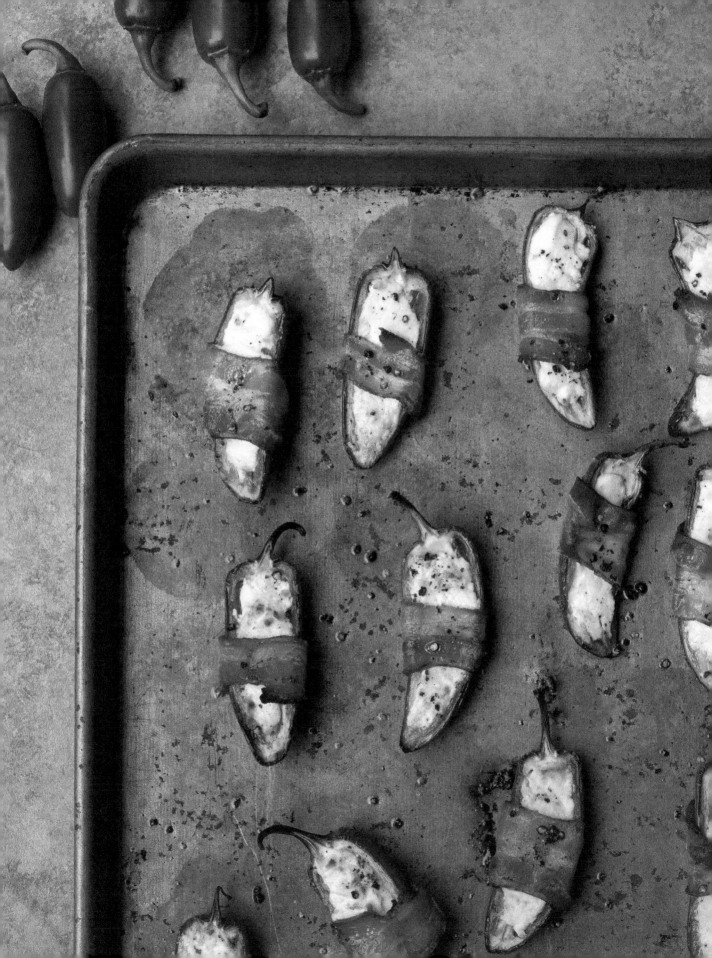

CHEESE ROLL-UPS

This recipe may be familiar to you—maybe your mom made it as an after-school snack when you were a kid. I like these because they're fast and easy and really delicious, plus I almost always have these ingredients in my refrigerator. Part of going keto means getting used to foods without the part you always thought held them together; in this case, it's a wrap without the wrap.

MAKES 4 ROLL-UPS

PREP TIME: 5 minutes
COOK TIME: 0 minutes

4 slices provolone cheese (circular ones work best)

8 slices deli turkey

3 to 4 tablespoons Keto Mayonnaise (page 225)

Salt

Freshly ground black pepper

PER SERVING (1 roll-up):
Calories: 189; Total carbs: 7g;
**Net carbs: 7g, 14%; Total fat: 12g, 54%;
Protein: 15g, 32%;** Fiber: 0g; Sugar: 3g

VARIATION 1: Calories: 146;
Total carbs: 4g; **Net carbs: 2g, 9%;
Total fat: 11g, 69%; Protein: 8g, 22%;**
Fiber: 2g; Sugar: 1g

VARIATION 2: Calories: 122;
Total carbs: 1g; **Net carbs: 1g, 4%;
Total fat: 9g, 67%; Protein: 9g, 29%;**
Fiber: 0g; Sugar: 0g

Lay out the provolone slices on a work surface. Layer 2 slices of turkey on each and add a smear of mayo. Season with salt and pepper and roll up like a wrap. Serve immediately.

VARIATION 1 **CHEESE VEGGIE ROLL-UPS:** Use Ranch Dressing (page 225) instead of mayo and layer thinly sliced green bell peppers and tomato on each slice of cheese. Roll up and serve.

VARIATION 2 **PEPPERONI PIZZA CHEESE ROLL-UPS:** Use pepperoni instead of turkey and pizza sauce instead of mayo.

KETO TACO SHELLS

For years I've been using lettuce leaves as taco shells for grain-free/low-carb tacos, but recently I decided to do a little experimenting to see if I could come up with something that has more crunch and mimics a corn tortilla in some ways. My brother-in-law makes cheesy taco shells in a pan on the stove, so I took his recipe and changed it so you can make them two at a time in the oven. It's a one-ingredient recipe that adds so much flavor and texture to keto tacos, I bet you'll never go back! **MAKES 4 SERVINGS**

PREP TIME: 5 minutes
COOK TIME: 20 minutes

6 ounces shredded cheese

PER SERVING (1 taco shell):
Calories: 168; Total carbs: 1g;
Net carbs: 1g, 2%; Total fat: 14g, 72%;
Protein: 11g, 26%; Fiber: 0g; Sugar: 0g

VARIATION 1: Calories: 339;
Total carbs: 5g; **Net carbs: 4g, 6%;**
Total fat: 18g, 47%; Protein: 39g, 47%;
Fiber: 1g; Sugar: 3g

VARIATION 2: Calories: 168;
Total carbs: 1g; **Net carbs: 1g, 2%;**
Total fat: 14g, 72%; Protein: 11g, 26%;
Fiber: 0g; Sugar: 0g

1. Preheat the oven to 350°F.

2. Line a baking sheet with a silicone baking mat or parchment paper.

3. Separate the cheese into 4 (1½-ounce) portions and make small circular piles a few inches apart (they will spread a bit in the oven). Pat the cheese down so all the piles are equally thick. Bake for 10 to 12 minutes or until the edges begin to brown. Cool for just a couple of minutes.

4. Lay a wooden spoon or spatula across two overturned glasses. Repeat to make a second setup, and carefully transfer a baked cheese circle to drape over the length of each spoon or spatula. Let them cool into the shape of a taco shell.

5. Fill with your choice of protein and top with chopped lettuce, avocado, salsa, sour cream, or whatever else you like on your tacos. These taco shells will keep refrigerated in an airtight container for a few days, but they are best freshly made and still a little warm.

VARIATION 1 **KETO SHREDDED CHICKEN TACOS:** Make shredded chicken in the slow cooker: Cook 1 pound boneless skinless chicken breasts or thighs on low heat for 8 hours with 1 jar of your favorite salsa. Shred the chicken with two forks and serve in the taco shells topped with sour cream, lettuce, and more salsa if desired.

VARIATION 2 **KETO TOSTADAS:** Skip step 4 and leave the taco shells flat to cool. Spread with sour cream and add your toppings, eating it like a tostada instead of a taco.

PERFECT PAIR: Top your tacos with Everyday Guacamole (page 38).

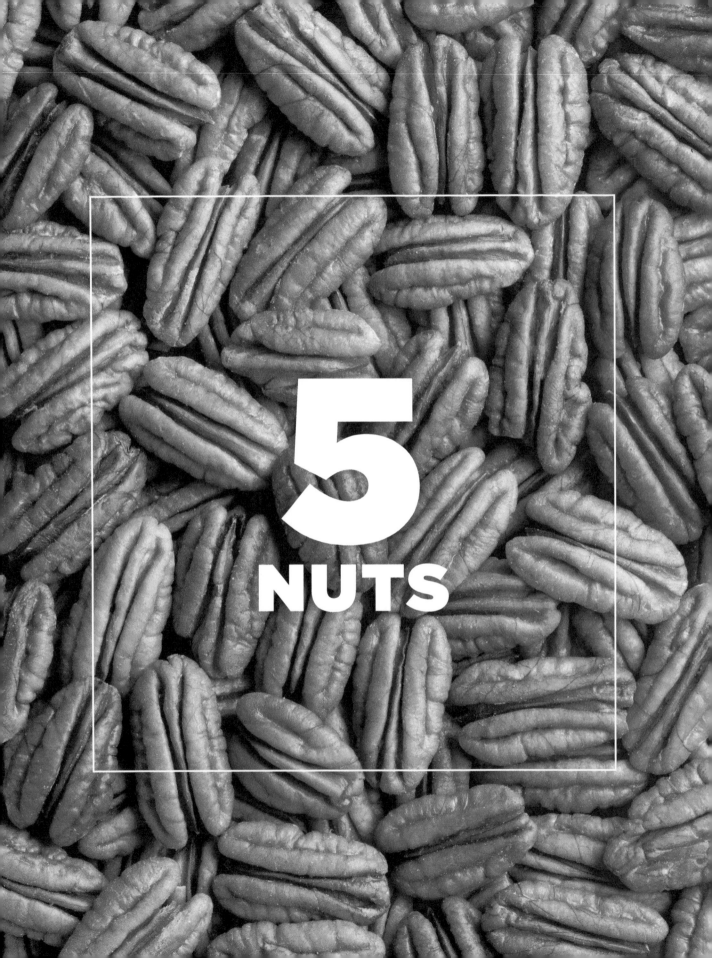

5
NUTS

Nuts are a great snack if you need a little protein, and there are lots of grain-free recipes that use nuts as a substitute for more conventional ingredients. That doesn't mean, however, that all nuts are keto-friendly. As usual, stick with the nuts that have the fewest carbs and the most fat. The majority of the recipes in this chapter use the lowest-carb nuts: pecans, hazelnuts, macadamia nuts, peanuts, and almonds. Other nuts (and seeds) that are low in carbs and therefore can be used as substitutes are Brazil nuts, chia seeds, sesame seeds, and walnuts.

The recipes here are mostly for snacks—Roasted Spiced Nut Mix (page 66), nut butter, Low-Carb Granola Bars (page 70), crackers, etc. I like to keep some nuts in my bag as an emergency snack, but that can get a little boring. These recipes ensure you always have snacks on hand that are delicious, interesting, and keto friendly.

EXTRA-KETO HOMEMADE NUT BUTTER

Do you know how easy it is to make your own nut butter? All you need is a few minutes, some nuts, and a food processor. I make my own and add some extra fat to make it even more keto-friendly. The easiest way to do this without adding any additional carbs or protein is just to add coconut oil—so that's what we're going to do here! **MAKES ABOUT 6 SERVINGS**

PREP TIME: 10 minutes
COOK TIME: 0 minutes

1 cup almonds, pecans, or macadamia nuts

¼ cup coconut oil

Pinch salt (optional)

PER SERVING (3 tablespoons):
Calories: 219; Total carbs: 5g;
**Net carbs: 2g, 9%; Total fat: 21g, 83%;
Protein: 5g, 8%;** Fiber: 3g; Sugar: 1g

VARIATION 1: Calories: 223;
Total carbs: 6g; **Net carbs: 3g, 9%;
Total fat: 22g, 82%; Protein: 6g, 9%;**
Fiber: 3g; Sugar: 1g

VARIATION 2: Calories: 224;
Total carbs: 5g; **Net carbs: 2g, 10%;
Total fat: 21g, 81%; Protein: 5g, 9%;**
Fiber: 3g; Sugar: 1g

1. In a food processor, process the nuts for 5 to 10 minutes or until they combine into a butter-like consistency and reach your desired smoothness. (I like mine completely smooth, but you can certainly leave it "crunchy.")

2. Add the coconut oil and process for 1 to 2 minutes more.

3. Add a pinch of salt (if using) and pulse to combine. Serve immediately. Refrigerate leftovers in an airtight container for up to 2 weeks.

VARIATION 1 **CHOCOLATE NUT BUTTER:** Add 1 to 2 tablespoons unsweetened cocoa powder when you add the coconut oil.

VARIATION 2 **VANILLA CINNAMON NUT BUTTER:** Add 2 teaspoons vanilla extract and 1 teaspoon ground cinnamon to the nut butter. Stir to combine.

BAKED BRIE WITH PECANS

One of my favorite treats around the holidays is baked Brie cheese. Unfortunately, it's usually wrapped in puff pastry and served with some kind of fruit jam on top, so there's nothing keto about it. I decided to make a low-carb baked Brie for this year's festivities, and it's a lot more straightforward. Topped with herbed pecans and a little olive oil, this baked Brie will be the star of your next potluck dinner or special-occasion party.

MAKES 6 SERVINGS

PREP TIME: 5 minutes
COOK TIME: 10 minutes

1 (¾-pound) wheel Brie cheese

3 ounces pecans, chopped

2 garlic cloves, minced

2 tablespoons minced fresh rosemary leaves

1½ tablespoons olive oil

Salt

Freshly ground black pepper

PER SERVING: Calories: 318;
Total carbs: 3g; **Net carbs: 2g, 4%;**
Total fat: 29g, 79%; Protein: 13g, 17%;
Fiber: 1g; Sugar: 1g

VARIATION 1: Calories: 244;
Total carbs: 1g; **Net carbs: 1g, 1%;**
Total fat: 20g, 74%; Protein: 15g, 25%;
Fiber: 0g; Sugar: 0g

VARIATION 2: Calories: 355;
Total carbs: 4g; **Net carbs: 2g, 4%;**
Total fat: 33g, 80%; Protein: 13g, 16%;
Fiber: 2g; Sugar: 1g

1. Preheat the oven to 400°F.

2. Line a baking sheet with parchment paper and place the Brie on it.

3. In a small bowl, stir together the pecans, garlic, rosemary, and olive oil. Season with salt and pepper. Spoon the mixture in an even layer over the Brie. Bake for about 10 minutes until the cheese is warm and the nuts are lightly browned.

4. Remove and let it cool for 1 to 2 minutes before serving.

VARIATION 1 **PROSCIUTTO-WRAPPED BAKED BRIE:** Wrap the cheese in 3 ounces thinly sliced prosciutto. Brush with 1 tablespoon olive oil and bake at 400°F for 10 minutes.

VARIATION 2 **BAKED BRIE WITH HERBED PECANS AND CARAMELIZED ONIONS:** Thinly slice ½ onion. Sauté it over low heat for 15 to 20 minutes in 2 tablespoons butter, stirring frequently, until golden brown and well caramelized. Top the Brie with the onions and top the onions with the nut mix from the recipe. Bake at 400°F for 10 minutes.

ROASTED SPICED NUT MIX

When we switched our diet to Paleo, my mom started making a spiced pecan snack that was so incredibly delicious—it had cinnamon and vanilla and some honey. This is a keto variation, using lots of butter and stevia instead of honey, although you could skip the sweetener altogether. I love eating these when they're still warm—something about the toasty flavors together with the cinnamon, vanilla, and butter just reminds me of a chilly fall afternoon and makes me want a cup of tea to go with it. **MAKES 8 SERVINGS**

PREP TIME: 10 minutes
COOK TIME: 10 minutes

 GF

1 teaspoon vanilla extract

1 teaspoon ground cinnamon

1 teaspoon ground allspice

½ teaspoon ground ginger

½ teaspoon ground nutmeg

1 teaspoon liquid stevia (optional)

4 tablespoons butter

1 cup pecans

½ cup almonds

½ cup macadamia nuts

PER SERVING (¼ cup): Calories: 279; Total carbs: 5g; **Net carbs: 2g, 7%; Total fat: 27g, 87%; Protein: 4g, 6%;** Fiber: 3g; Sugar: 1g

VARIATION 1: Calories: 279; Total carbs: 5g; **Net carbs: 2g, 7%; Total fat: 27g, 87%; Protein: 4g, 6%;** Fiber: 3g; Sugar: 1g

VARIATION 2: Calories: 279; Total carbs: 5g; **Net carbs: 2g, 7%; Total fat: 27g, 87%; Protein: 4g, 6%;** Fiber: 3g; Sugar: 1g

1. Preheat the oven to 375°F.

2. In a small bowl, combine the vanilla, cinnamon, allspice, ginger, nutmeg, and stevia (if using). Set aside.

3. In a large nonstick skillet over medium-low heat, melt the butter.

4. Add the pecans, almonds, and macadamias. Sprinkle the spice mixture over the nuts and stir to combine, ensuring the nuts are thoroughly coated in butter and spices. Cook for about 10 minutes or until the nuts are golden brown. Remove from the heat and cool slightly before serving.

5. Store in an airtight container on the counter for a few days or refrigerate for up to 1 week.

VARIATION 1 **OVEN-ROASTED SPICED NUT MIX:** Melt the butter in the microwave. Place the nuts on a rimmed baking sheet. Pour the melted butter over the nuts, sprinkle on the vanilla, spices, and stevia (if using), and toss to combine. Give the baking sheet a gentle shake to make sure the nuts are in an even layer. Bake at 375°F for about 15 minutes or until golden brown (keep an eye on them; they can go from almost done to burnt very quickly). Cool slightly and serve warm.

VARIATION 2 **SPICY ROASTED NUT MIX:** Instead of baking spices, season the nuts with 1 teaspoon garlic powder, some salt and pepper, and ½ teaspoon ground cayenne pepper. Follow the rest of the recipe as written.

ALMOND SESAME CRACKERS

My mom makes these Paleo crackers with almond flour. They're really simple but so delicious. It's great to have a crunchy snack that isn't full of preservatives and unnecessary ingredients, and these are keto-friendly as well! Try them with some turkey, cheese, and sliced veggies as a quick lunch or snack.

MAKES ABOUT 36 (1-INCH-SQUARE) CRACKERS

PREP TIME: 15 minutes
COOK TIME: 15 minutes

1½ cups almond flour

1 egg

3 tablespoons sesame seeds, divided

Salt

Freshly ground black pepper

PER SERVING (10 crackers): Calories: 108; Total carbs: 3g; **Net carbs: 1g, 11%; Total fat: 9g, 72%; Protein: 5g, 17%;** Fiber: 2g; Sugar: 0g

VARIATION 1: Calories: 102; Total carbs: 2g; **Net carbs: 1g, 11%; Total fat: 7g, 64%; Protein: 6g, 25%;** Fiber: 1g; Sugar: 1g

VARIATION 2: Calories: 109; Total carbs: 3g; **Net carbs: 1g, 11%; Total fat: 9g, 72%; Protein: 5g, 17%;** Fiber: 2g; Sugar: 0g

1. Preheat the oven to 350°F.

2. Line a baking sheet with parchment paper.

3. In a large bowl, mix together the almond flour, egg, and 1½ tablespoons of sesame seeds. Transfer the dough to a sheet of parchment and pat it out flat with your clean hands. Cover with another piece of parchment paper and roll it into a large square, at least 10 inches wide.

4. Remove the top piece of parchment and use a pizza cutter or sharp knife to cut the dough into small squares, about 1 inch wide. Season with salt and pepper and sprinkle with the remaining 1½ tablespoons of sesame seeds.

5. Remove the crackers from the parchment and place them on the prepared baking sheet. Bake for about 15 minutes or until the crackers begin to brown. Cool before serving, and store any leftovers in an airtight bag or container on your counter for up to 2 weeks.

VARIATION 1 GARLIC PARMESAN CRACKERS: Skip the sesame seeds and add 1 tablespoon garlic powder to the dough. Sprinkle the crackers with ¼ cup grated Parmesan before baking.

VARIATION 2 HERBED ALMOND CRACKERS: Add 1 teaspoon dried basil, 1 teaspoon dried oregano, and 1 teaspoon dried rosemary to the cracker dough. Follow the rest of the recipe as written.

GREEN BEANS ALMONDINE

Buttery green beans with a little lemon juice are one of my favorite side dishes, but when topped with toasty slivered almonds they're just the best. The green beans cook really fast, as do the almonds, so make them simultaneously and have this dish ready to serve in no time. **MAKES 4 SERVINGS**

PREP TIME: 10 minutes
COOK TIME: 10 minutes

1 pound green beans, rinsed and trimmed

¼ cup slivered almonds

2 tablespoons butter

1 tablespoon freshly squeezed lemon juice

Salt

Freshly ground black pepper

PER SERVING: Calories: 163;
Total carbs: 11g; **Net carbs:5 g, 26%;**
Total fat: 13g, 65%; Protein: 5g, 9%;
Fiber: 6g; Sugar: 2g

VARIATION 1: Calories: 227;
Total carbs: 13g; **Net carbs: 7g, 21%;**
Total fat: 18g, 70%; Protein: 7g, 9%;
Fiber: 6g; Sugar: 3g

VARIATION 2: Calories: 253;
Total carbs: 3g; **Net carbs: 1g, 5%;**
Total fat: 19g, 65%; Protein: 18g, 30%;
Fiber: 2g; Sugar: 1g

1. Bring a large saucepan of water to a boil over high heat. Add the green beans. Cook for 5 to 7 minutes or until the beans are bright green and tender but not soft or soggy.

2. While the beans cook, in a small skillet over medium-low heat, melt the butter, add the almonds, and cook them for 3 to 4 minutes until golden brown and fragrant. Remove from the heat and stir in the lemon juice. Season with salt and pepper.

3. Drain the beans and pour the lemony, buttery almonds over them. Season again with salt and pepper, if needed. Serve immediately. Refrigerate leftovers in an airtight container for up to 5 days.

VARIATION 1 **BRUSSELS SPROUTS ALMONDINE:** Quarter 1 pound Brussels sprouts. Sauté them with 2 tablespoons butter in a large skillet over medium heat for about 10 minutes or until fork-tender. Transfer to a serving bowl. Return the pan to the heat and add the almonds, more butter, and the lemon juice. Pour over the sprouts and serve.

VARIATION 2 **SOLE ALMONDINE:** Make this a main dish by pouring the lemony buttered almonds over some fish: panfry 2 sole fillets in 1 tablespoon butter over medium heat for 3 to 4 minutes per side and serve with the almonds on top.

LOW-CARB GRANOLA BARS

Finding keto-friendly snacks to take with you on the go can be a challenge. I would say that the ultimate keto snack is a hardboiled egg, but these low-carb granola bars are a little more of a treat, so you can mix it up every now and then. **MAKES ABOUT 12 BARS**

PREP TIME: 10 minutes
COOK TIME: 15 to 20 minutes

1 cup almonds

1 cup hazelnuts

1 cup unsweetened coconut flakes

1 egg

¼ cup coconut oil, melted

¼ cup unsweetened peanut butter

½ cup dark chocolate chips

1 tablespoon vanilla extract

1 tablespoon ground cinnamon

Pinch salt

PER SERVING (1 bar): Calories: 588; Total carbs: 6g; **Net carbs: 5g, 5%; Total fat: 58g, 87%; Protein: 11g, 8%;** Fiber: 1g; Sugar: 5g

VARIATION 1: Calories: 271; Total carbs: 10g; **Net carbs: 6g, 13%; Total fat: 25g, 84%; Protein: 5g, 3%;** Fiber: 4g; Sugar: 3g

VARIATION 2: Calories: 272; Total carbs: 10g; **Net carbs: 6g, 13%; Total fat: 25g, 84%; Protein: 5g, 3%;** Fiber: 4g; Sugar: 5g

1. Preheat the oven to 350°F.

2. In a food processor, pulse together the almonds and macadamia nuts for 1 to 2 minutes until roughly chopped. (You want them pretty fine but not turning into nut butter.) Transfer them to a large bowl.

3. Stir in the coconut, egg, coconut oil, peanut butter, chocolate chips, vanilla, cinnamon, and salt. Transfer the mixture to an 8- or 9-inch square baking dish and gently press into an even layer. Bake for 15 to 20 minutes or until golden brown. Cool and cut into 12 bars. Refrigerate in an airtight container for up to 2 weeks.

VARIATION 1 **LOW-CARB CHOCOLATE GRANOLA BARS:**
Add 2 tablespoons unsweetened cocoa powder to the bar mix.

VARIATION 2 **LOW-CARB RASPBERRY GRANOLA BARS:**
If you have room for extra carbs and want to add some fruit, stir in ½ cup chopped fresh raspberries.

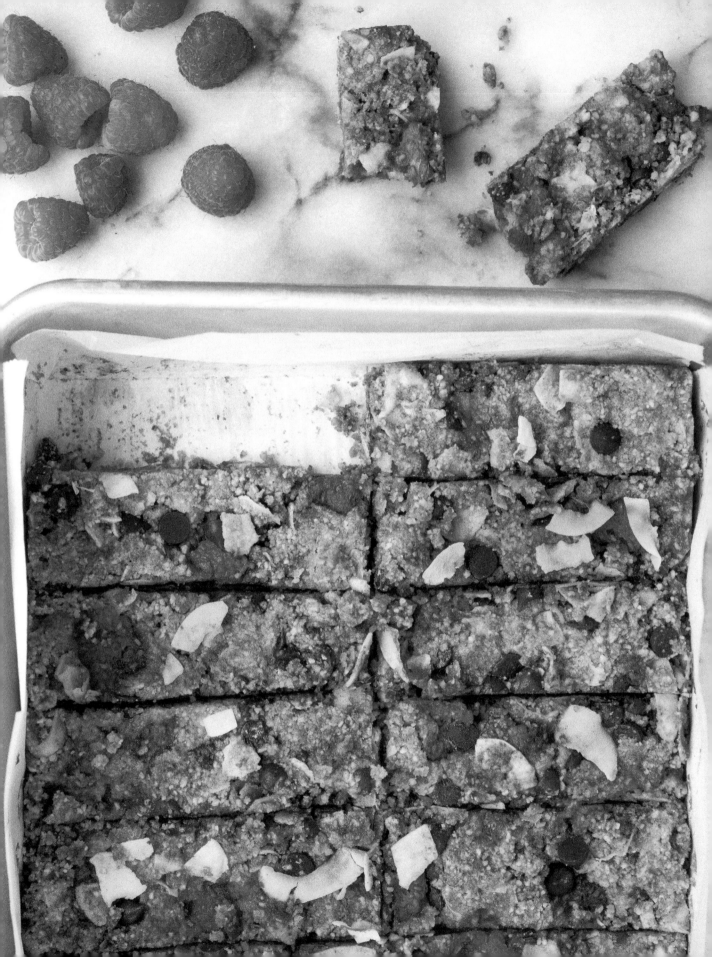

PEANUT BUTTER KETO FUDGE

This fudge is truly decadent and easy to make; people will be so impressed you made it from scratch *and* managed to keep it low-carb. Add some stevia or other low-carb sweetener if you like, but I've found that once you get keto adapted, you really don't crave sweetness anymore, and the richness of the peanut butter with the cream cheese ends up being perfectly satisfying.

MAKES 12 SERVINGS

PREP TIME: 5 minutes
COOK TIME: 10 minutes
CHILLING TIME: 1 hour

½ cup (1 stick) butter

8 ounces cream cheese

1 cup unsweetened peanut butter

1 teaspoon vanilla extract (or the seeds from 1 vanilla bean)

1 teaspoon liquid stevia (optional)

PER SERVING (1 fudge square):
Calories: 261; Total carbs: 5g;
**Net carbs: 4g, 4%; Total fat: 24g, 83%;
Protein: 8g, 12%;** Fiber: 1g; Sugar: 2g

VARIATION 1: Calories: 261;
Total carbs: 5g; **Net carbs: 4g, 4%;
Total fat: 24g, 83%; Protein: 8g, 12%;**
Fiber: 1g; Sugar: 2g

VARIATION 2: Calories: 288;
Total carbs: 7g; **Net carbs: 4g, 6%;
Total fat: 27g, 83%; Protein: 9g, 11%;**
Fiber: 3g; Sugar: 2g

1. Line an 8- or 9-inch square or 9-by-13-inch rectangular baking dish with parchment paper. Set aside.

2. In a saucepan over medium heat, melt the butter and cream cheese together, stirring frequently, for about 5 minutes.

3. Add the peanut butter and continue to stir until smooth. Remove from the heat.

4. Stir in the vanilla and stevia (if using). Pour the mixture into the prepared dish and spread into an even layer. Refrigerate for about 1 hour until thickened and set enough to cut and handle. Cut into small squares and enjoy! Refrigerate, covered, for up to 1 week.

VARIATION 1 **CHOCOLATE HAZELNUT KETO FUDGE:** Make hazelnut butter following the Extra-Keto Homemade Nut Butter recipe (page 64) and use it instead of the peanut butter. Add 2 to 3 tablespoons unsweetened cocoa powder and follow the rest of the recipe as written.

VARIATION 2 **DARK CHOCOLATE KETO FUDGE:** Add 2 ounces unsweetened baking chocolate to the pan to melt with the cream cheese and butter. Add ¼ cup unsweetened cocoa powder, stir well to combine, and follow the rest of the recipe from step 3.

KETO CHEESECAKE WITH HAZELNUT CRUST

One thing I have really enjoyed about experimenting with keto is being able to incorporate dairy into my diet on a regular basis again—that means cream in my coffee and cheese on my eggs, but it also means cheesecake! Once you go sugar-free I think you'll find that less sweet desserts are just as satisfying, so this lightly sweetened pie with hazelnut crust should do the trick every time.

MAKES 10 SERVINGS

PREP TIME: 10 minutes
COOK TIME: 1 hour 45 minutes
CHILLING TIME: 3 hours or overnight

4 tablespoons butter, melted, plus more for the pan

1 cup finely crushed hazelnuts

1 cup almond flour

5 (8-ounce) blocks cream cheese, at room temperature

1½ cups Swerve

4 eggs

1 teaspoon vanilla extract

1 cup sour cream

PER SERVING: Calories: 578; Total carbs: 7g; **Net carbs: 6g, 5%; Total fat: 58g, 87%; Protein: 12g, 8%;** Fiber: 1g; Sugar: 5g

VARIATION 1: Calories: 591; Total carbs: 10g; **Net carbs: 7g, 5%; Total fat: 59g, 87%; Protein: 12g, 8%;** Fiber: 3g; Sugar: 5g

VARIATION 2: Calories: 583; Total carbs: 8g; **Net carbs: 7g, 5%; Total fat: 58g, 87%; Protein: 11g, 8%;** Fiber: 1g; Sugar: 5g

1. Preheat the oven to 375°F.

2. Grease a 10-inch springform pan with melted butter.

3. In a large bowl, stir together the hazelnuts and almond flour. Pour the melted butter over them and stir until the nut mixture becomes wet and crumbly. Scrape the crust into the prepared pan, pressing firmly with your fingers. Bake for about 15 minutes or until the crust begins to brown. Remove from the oven and let it cool completely.

4. Reduce the oven temperature to 325°F.

5. In a bowl, beat the cream cheese with a handheld mixer until fluffy. Continue to beat as you add the Swerve.

6. Add the eggs one at a time, beating well after each addition.

7. Continue to beat while adding the vanilla followed by the sour cream.

8. Fill a large deeply rimmed baking sheet halfway with hot water. Carefully transfer the springform pan with the crust to the water bath and pour the cheesecake filling into the crust. Bake for 1 hour, 30 minutes or until you can slide a knife in and it comes out clean. Let the cheesecake cool then refrigerate for several hours, preferably overnight.

VARIATION 1 **CHOCOLATE CHEESECAKE:** Add ½ cup unsweetened cocoa powder to the cheesecake filling after adding the eggs.

VARIATION 2 **LEMON CHEESECAKE:** Add the juice of 1½ lemons to the cheesecake mix instead of the vanilla. Serve garnished with thinly sliced lemons.

LEMON BARS WITH CASHEW CRUST

These lemon bars are tart and refreshing with a rich, buttery cashew crust. The recipe basically reads like a lemon fat bomb recipe combined with a nut crust, but the finished product reminds me so much of lemon bars from a conventional bakery. **MAKES 12 BARS**

PREP TIME: 5 minutes
COOK TIME: 35 minutes

2 tablespoons butter, melted, plus 2 tablespoons, at room temperature, plus more for the baking dish

1 cup finely crushed cashews

1 cup almond flour

½ cup Swerve

Zest of 2 lemons

½ cup freshly squeezed lemon juice

6 egg yolks

2 tablespoons gelatin

PER SERVING (1 bar): Calories: 144; Total carbs: 4g; **Net carbs: 4g, 11%; Total fat: 13g, 78%; Protein: 4g, 11%;** Fiber: 0g; Sugar: 1g

VARIATION 1: Calories: 145; Total carbs: 4g; **Net carbs: 3g, 11%; Total fat: 13g, 78%; Protein: 4g, 11%;** Fiber: 1g; Sugar: 1g

VARIATION 2: Calories: 169; Total carbs: 5g; **Net carbs: 4g, 11%; Total fat: 15g, 79%; Protein: 4g, 10%;** Fiber: 1g; Sugar: 1g

1. Preheat the oven to 375°F.

2. Grease an 8- or 9-inch square baking dish with butter.

3. In a large bowl, stir together the cashews and almond flour. Pour the melted butter over them and stir until the nut mixture becomes wet and crumbly. Scrape the crust into the prepared dish, pressing down firmly with your fingers. Bake for about 15 minutes or until the crust begins to brown. Remove from the oven and let it cool completely.

4. Reduce the oven temperature to 350°F.

5. In a small saucepan over low heat, melt the 2 tablespoons of room-temperature butter.

6. Stir in the Swerve, lemon zest, and lemon juice.

7. Slowly add the egg yolks one at a time, whisking to incorporate as the filling thickens. Cook for 2 to 3 minutes, whisking.

8. Remove from the heat and whisk in the gelatin until the mixture is smooth. Pour the lemon filling over the crust and spread it evenly. Bake for 10 to 12 minutes. Remove it from the oven and let it cool. Cut into 12 squares and serve. Refrigerate, covered, for up to 1 week.

VARIATION 1 **RASPBERRY LEMON BARS:** Top these bars with ¼ cup chopped fresh raspberries.

VARIATION 2 **COCONUT LEMON BARS:** When the lemon bars come out of the oven, top with ½ cup unsweetened shredded coconut.

SALTED CHOCOLATE-MACADAMIA NUT FAT BOMBS

Fat bombs are my favorite keto treat. Chocolate, almond butter, coconut oil—what's not to love? These particular bombs are especially delicious because they combine salted chocolate with crushed macadamia nuts and truly taste like dessert. I like to use a little grass-fed butter in mine for extra richness, but you could just stick to coconut oil if you like. **MAKES 5 SERVINGS**

PREP TIME: 10 minutes
COOK TIME: 10 minutes
CHILLING TIME: 15 to 20 minutes

½ cup coconut oil

½ cup almond butter

¼ cup unsweetened cocoa powder

1 to 2 tablespoons butter (optional)

Pinch salt

¼ cup chopped macadamia nuts

PER SERVING (1 bomb):
Calories: 443; Total carbs: 9g;
Net carbs: 6g, 6%; Total fat: 47g, 90%;
Protein: 5g, 4%; Fiber: 3g; Sugar: 0g

VARIATION 1: Calories: 433;
Total carbs: 9g; **Net carbs: 6g, 7%;**
Total fat: 45g, 89%; Protein: 5g, 4%;
Fiber: 3g; Sugar: 1g

VARIATION 2: Calories: 443;
Total carbs: 9g; **Net carbs: 6g, 6%;**
Total fat: 47g, 90%; Protein: 5g, 4%;
Fiber: 3g; Sugar: 0g

1. In a small saucepan over low heat, melt the coconut oil.

2. Whisk in the almond butter until well combined.

3. Add the cocoa powder and butter (if using). Continue to whisk until combined.

4. Add the salt, remove the pan from the heat, and give it one more stir. Cool slightly before pouring the mixture into a mold—use silicone cupcake liners, a cocktail ice-cube tray, or even muffin tins with paper or silicone liners. Top with the macadamia nuts.

5. Freeze for 15 to 20 minutes or until they've hardened enough to handle. Refrigerate leftovers in an airtight container for up to 2 weeks.

VARIATION 1 **COCONUT ALMOND FAT BOMBS:** Instead of macadamia nuts, top with unsweetened shredded coconut.

VARIATION 2 **FAT BOMB CHOCOLATE BARK:** Pour the mixture onto a parchment paper-lined baking sheet instead of into molds. Freeze for 15 to 20 minutes and chop into chocolate bark. Keep refrigerated.

6
CHICKEN

ost health-conscious diets sing chicken's praises for being high in protein and low in fat. For a ketogenic diet, however, chicken is sometimes a little *too* high in protein without enough fat, so a lot of these recipes have fat added in some way. Most of the chicken recipes call for chicken breasts, but just go right for the thighs if you prefer. I usually choose them because they're fattier, tastier, less expensive, and harder to overcook.

This chapter has a lot of dinner recipes, some salads, and my all-time favorite recipe, Buffalo Chicken Dip (page 78). I've also included my Easy Marinated Chicken Thighs (page 89), which I make at least once a week. Grilled chicken thighs with some salad greens on the side dressed simply with Ranch Dressing (page 225) is one of the easiest meals to throw together and always tasty. I hope these recipes give you lots of inspiration for using chicken in new ways!

BUFFALO CHICKEN DIP

I made this dip for our first keto Super Bowl. We wanted something to munch during the game that felt football-y, but we didn't want to stray from our low-carb, high-fat diet. This recipe is perfect because all the dairy you add to the chicken ups the fat content. And the best part is that it all comes together easily in a slow cooker. **MAKES 8 SERVINGS**

PREP TIME: 10 minutes
COOK TIME: 4 to 6 hours

1 pound boneless skinless chicken breasts

8 ounces full-fat cream cheese

4 ounces crumbled blue cheese

2 cups shredded mozzarella cheese

1 cup Frank's RedHot Sauce

1 cup sour cream

4 scallions, green parts only, sliced

Carrot sticks, sliced (optional)

Celery sticks, sliced (optional)

PER SERVING: Calories: 298;
Total carbs: 4g; **Net carbs: 4g, 6%;**
Total fat: 22g, 66%; Protein: 21g, 28%;
Fiber: 0g; Sugar: 1g

VARIATION 1: Calories: 390;
Total carbs: 4g; **Net carbs: 4g, 3%;**
Total fat: 30g, 70%; Protein: 26g, 27%;
Fiber: 0g; Sugar: 1g

VARIATION 2: Calories: 298;
Total carbs: 4g; **Net carbs: 4g, 6%;**
Total fat: 22g, 66%; Protein: 21g, 28%;
Fiber: 0g; Sugar: 1g

1. Place the chicken breasts in the slow cooker. Cook for 2 to 3 hours on low heat (or on high heat for about 1 hour). When the chicken is cooked, remove it from the slow cooker and dice, shred, or chop it roughly. Return it to the slow cooker.

2. Add the cream cheese, blue cheese, mozzarella, hot sauce, and sour cream. Stir well with a spatula to combine everything. Cook on low heat for 2 to 3 hours more or until everything is melted and heated through. Top with the scallions and serve with sliced veggies (carrots and celery are my favorites with this), if desired.

VARIATION 1 **BUFFALO CHICKEN DIP WITH CHEDDAR:** Use shredded Cheddar cheese instead of the mozzarella.

VARIATION 2 **OVEN-BAKED BUFFALO CHICKEN DIP:** If you don't have a slow cooker, mix the cooked chicken with the remaining ingredients in a baking dish. Bake at 350°F for about 20 minutes or until heated through.

MAKE AHEAD: Cook the chicken breasts a day or two ahead and cut down on some of the time this recipe takes. You can also make the entire recipe ahead of time, reheat in the microwave for 2 to 3 minutes, and transfer to the slow cooker on low heat until ready to serve.

KETO CHICKEN STRIPS

These keto chicken strips are great because when you're eating low-carb, sometimes you just need a protein that's got some crunch to it—but breading or batter or any kind is pretty much always a no-go. With a little egg wash and some almond flour, you can quickly and easily create a keto-friendly breading for chicken tenders that does the trick! **MAKES 4 SERVINGS**

PREP TIME: 10 minutes
COOK TIME: 35 minutes

Olive oil, or butter, for preparing the baking sheet

1½ pounds boneless skinless chicken breasts, cut into 12 strips

Salt

Freshly ground black pepper

2 eggs

1 cup almond flour

PER SERVING: Calories: 253; Total carbs: 0g; **Net carbs: 0g, 1%;** **Total fat: 8g, 28%; Protein: 42g, 71%;** Fiber: 0g; Sugar: 0g

VARIATION 1: Calories: 303; Total carbs: 0g; **Net carbs: 0g, 1%;** **Total fat: 14g, 59%; Protein: 43g, 59%;** Fiber: 0g; Sugar: 0g

VARIATION 2: Calories: 258; Total carbs: 1g; **Net carbs: 1g, 2%;** **Total fat: 8g, 28%; Protein: 43g, 70%;** Fiber: 0g; Sugar: 1g

1. Preheat the oven to 350°F.

2. Lightly grease a baking sheet with olive oil and set aside.

3. Season the chicken strips with salt and pepper.

4. Break the eggs into a shallow dish and whisk to combine.

5. Place the almond flour in a separate shallow dish and season with more salt and pepper.

6. Dip each piece of chicken first into the eggs and then into the almond flour. Flip the chicken to ensure the whole piece is coated with almond flour. Place the strips on the prepared baking sheet and bake for about 30 minutes until lightly browned and cooked through (the juices will run clear).

7. Turn the oven to broil, and broil the chicken for 1 to 2 minutes to get them nicely browned. Serve immediately. Refrigerate leftovers in an airtight container for up to 5 days. Reheat for 1 minute in the microwave, or in the oven at 350°F for 15 to 20 minutes.

VARIATION 1 **BUFFALO CHICKEN STRIPS:** After cooking, toss the chicken strips in a 1:1 ratio of 2 tablespoons melted butter and 2 tablespoons Frank's RedHot Sauce, or serve it on the side as a dipping sauce.

VARIATION 2 **CAJUN CHICKEN STRIPS:** Season the almond flour with Cajun spice mix—mix together 1 teaspoon salt, 1 teaspoon garlic powder, 1 teaspoon paprika, 1 teaspoon freshly ground black pepper, and 1 teaspoon ground cayenne pepper.

PERFECT PAIR: These chicken strips are delicious with a side of Ranch Dressing (page 225) for dipping.

KETO CHICKEN SALAD

This chicken salad may look familiar if you've already made my Chicken Salad–Stuffed Avocados (page 42). Chicken salad is easy to make in large quantities and use throughout the week. My favorite way to make it is usually with lots of grapes, but as they're high in carbs this recipe calls for just a few—one serving has about 2 carbs from the fruit. **MAKES 4 SERVINGS**

PREP TIME: 10 minutes
COOK TIME: 0 minutes

1 (12.5-ounce) can chicken, drained

½ cup Keto Mayonnaise (page 225)

½ celery stalk, diced

1 scallion, green parts only, thinly sliced

½ cup grapes, finely diced

Salt

Freshly ground black pepper

PER SERVING: Calories: 291;
Total carbs: 12g; **Net carbs: 12g, 15%;**
Total fat: 17g, 52%; Protein: 23g, 33%;
Fiber: 0g; Sugar: 5g

VARIATION 1: Calories: 283;
Total carbs: 9g; **Net carbs: 8g, 12%;**
Total fat: 17g, 54%; Protein: 23g, 34%;
Fiber: 1g; Sugar: 2g

VARIATION 2: Calories: 297;
Total carbs: 13g; **Net carbs: 12g, 16%;**
Total fat: 17g, 51%; Protein: 23g, 33%;
Fiber: 1g; Sugar: 6g

In a large bowl, combine the chicken, mayonnaise, celery, scallion, and grapes. Season with salt and pepper and stir until combined. Serve immediately or refrigerate in an airtight container for up to 5 days.

VARIATION 1 **CURRY CHICKEN SALAD:** Skip the grapes and add 1 tablespoon curry powder to the salad. Stir well.

VARIATION 2 **CUCUMBER DILL CHICKEN SALAD:** Add ½ cucumber, finely diced, and about 2 tablespoons chopped fresh dill to the chicken salad. Squeeze the juice of ½ lemon over everything and stir well to combine.

COBB SALAD

If I'm out and about and need to grab a quick, healthy lunch that won't throw off my macros, I always opt for a Cobb salad. There's a place in Palo Alto that makes great salads and their Cobb is my favorite. Grilled chicken, bacon, blue cheese, avocado, and fresh, crisp lettuce—hungry? It's seriously one of the most perfect keto salads. **MAKES 1 SERVING**

PREP TIME: 10 minutes
COOK TIME: 0 minutes

½ head romaine lettuce, chopped

4 ounces grilled chicken breast, chopped or sliced

½ avocado, diced

1 hardboiled egg, sliced

2 bacon slices, cooked and crumbled

1 ounce crumbled blue cheese

¼ cup Ranch Dressing (page 225)

Salt

Freshly ground black pepper

PER SERVING: Calories: 831;
Total carbs: 24g; **Net carbs: 22g, 11%;**
Total fat: 53g, 58%; Protein: 64g, 31%;
Fiber: 2g; Sugar: 5g

VARIATION 1: Calories: 1087;
Total carbs: 22g; **Net carbs: 20g, 9%;**
Total fat: 81g, 67%; Protein: 64g, 24%;
Fiber: 2g; Sugar: 5g

VARIATION 2: Calories: 781;
Total carbs: 21g; **Net carbs: 19g, 12%;**
Total fat: 47g, 54%; Protein: 64g, 24%;
Fiber: 2g; Sugar: 5g

1. In a large bowl, combine the lettuce, chicken, avocado, egg, bacon, and blue cheese.

2. Add the dressing and toss well to combine, ensuring the entire salad is dressed. Season with salt and pepper and serve immediately.

VARIATION 1 **COBB SALAD WITH RED WINE VINAIGRETTE:** Instead of ranch dressing, toss this salad with 2 tablespoons olive oil, 2 tablespoons red wine vinegar, and 1 teaspoon Dijon mustard (whisked together in a small bowl before adding to the salad).

VARIATION 2 **COBB SALAD WITH CHEDDAR CHEESE:** If you aren't a fan of blue cheese, substitute shredded or cubed Cheddar.

CHICKEN CAESAR SALAD

Caesar salads were never a favorite of mine when I was growing up, but as an adult I've changed my tune. I love most of the components of a chicken Caesar salad: crisp romaine lettuce, peppery Parmesan cheese, fresh lemon juice . . . basically I love all of it except the anchovy. But this dressing uses anchovy sparingly and it all comes together so nicely that I make this salad regularly, especially if I'm having friends over for lunch or dinner. **MAKES 1 SERVING**

PREP TIME: 15 minutes
COOK TIME: 0 minutes

¼ cup olive oil

1 garlic clove

1 anchovy fillet, finely chopped

Juice of ½ lemon

Salt

Freshly ground black pepper

4 ounces grilled chicken breast, chopped or sliced

½ large head romaine lettuce, chopped

¼ cup grated Parmesan cheese

PER SERVING: Calories: 817; Total carbs: 16g; **Net carbs: 15g, 10%;** **Total fat: 61g, 67%; Protein: 47g, 23%;** Fiber: 1g; Sugar: 9g

VARIATION 1: Calories: 943; Total carbs: 18g; **Net carbs: 17g, 6%;** **Total fat: 63g, 61%; Protein: 72g, 31%;** Fiber: 1g; Sugar: 9g

VARIATION 2: Calories: 837; Total carbs: 20g; **Net carbs: 17g, 11%;** **Total fat: 61g, 66%; Protein: 48g, 23%;** Fiber: 3g; Sugar: 11g

1. In a blender, purée the olive oil, garlic, anchovy, and lemon juice to make the dressing. Season with salt and pepper.

2. In a large bowl, combine the chicken and romaine lettuce.

3. Add the dressing and toss to combine. Sprinkle with the Parmesan. Serve immediately.

VARIATION 1 **CAESAR SALAD WITH SHRIMP:** Omit the chicken and use 4 ounces cooked shrimp instead.

VARIATION 2 **CHICKEN CAESAR SALAD WITH ASPARAGUS:** Add an extra veggie to this dish by including 4 steamed asparagus spears, chopped.

KETO CHICKEN CORDON BLEU

This dish is really easy to make keto friendly—all you have to do is skip the bread crumbs! I remember always being so impressed by Chicken Cordon Bleu until I learned it was basically chicken rolled up with ham and cheese inside. But even knowing that, there's still something special about it. The flavors are wonderful together, and the Swiss cheese melts and bubbles and becomes this sumptuous new thing with smoky ham and juicy chicken. **MAKES 4 SERVINGS**

PREP TIME: 10 minutes
COOK TIME: 35 minutes

½ cup almond flour

Salt

Freshly ground black pepper

4 (4- to 6-ounce) boneless skinless chicken breasts

4 slices cooked ham

4 slices Swiss cheese

PER SERVING: Calories: 358;
Total carbs: 2g; **Net carbs: 2g, 2%;**
Total fat: 14g, 34%; Protein: 53g, 64%;
Fiber: 0g; Sugar: 0g

VARIATION 1: Calories: 565;
Total carbs: 2g; **Net carbs: 2g, 2%;**
Total fat: 37g, 58%; Protein: 54g, 40%;
Fiber:0 g; Sugar:0 g

VARIATION 2: Calories: 365;
Total carbs: 1g; **Net carbs: 1g, 1%;**
Total fat: 15g, 37%; Protein: 53g, 62%;
Fiber: 0g; Sugar: 0g

1. Preheat the oven to 350°F.

2. In a small bowl, season the almond flour with salt and pepper. Set aside.

3. Cover the chicken breasts with plastic wrap and pound them out to about ¼ inch thick. Season both sides with salt and pepper.

4. Layer 1 slice of ham and 1 slice of cheese on each piece of chicken. Roll each up as tightly as possible, securing with a toothpick.

5. Dust each rolled-up piece of chicken with seasoned almond flour and transfer to a baking dish just large enough to hold them in a single layer. Bake for about 30 minutes or until the chicken is cooked through and the juices run clear.

6. Turn the oven to broil and broil the chicken for about 2 minutes until nice and brown. Refrigerate leftovers in an airtight container for up to 5 days. Reheat in a 350°F oven for 15 to 20 minutes.

VARIATION 1 **CHICKEN CORDON BLEU WITH BACON:** Use cooked bacon instead of ham, about 2 pieces per chicken breast.

VARIATION 2 **CHICKEN CORDON BLEU WITH CHEDDAR:** Use sliced Cheddar instead of Swiss cheese.

CHICKEN BACON RANCH CASSEROLE

This casserole is a wonderful comfort food—it's cheesy and delicious, and what's not to love about chicken, bacon, and ranch together? I like to make it with precooked chicken because when the chicken is cooked at the same time and in the same pan as the bacon, the dish gets a little too greasy. Instead I just steam or boil the chicken, or cook it in the slow cooker for 2 to 3 hours on high heat, then shred it and refrigerate until ready to use.

MAKES 4 SERVINGS

PREP TIME: 15 minutes
COOK TIME: 35 minutes

4 bacon slices, chopped

¼ white onion, diced

1 garlic clove, minced

1 pound shredded cooked chicken (boneless skinless breasts or thighs)

3 tablespoons ranch seasoning (see spices in Ranch Dressing, page 225)

½ cup heavy (whipping) cream

2 eggs

1 cup shredded Cheddar cheese, divided

Salt

Freshly ground black pepper

1. Preheat the oven to 350°F.

2. In a medium nonstick skillet over medium heat, cook the bacon for about 5 minutes.

3. Add the onion and garlic. Cook for 5 to 7 minutes until the onion is softened and translucent. Remove the skillet from the heat and transfer the bacon-onion mixture to a large bowl, leaving behind most of the bacon fat in the skillet.

4. To the bowl, add the chicken and ranch seasoning. Stir well to combine, making sure everything is coated in the spices. Transfer to a 9-by-13-inch baking dish.

5. In the same bowl, whisk the cream and eggs. Add ½ cup of Cheddar, season with salt and pepper, and whisk to combine. Pour the cheese sauce over the chicken mixture and tap the baking dish on the counter to make sure the cheese sauce covers everything and makes it all the way to the bottom and sides of the dish. Top with the remaining ½ cup of Cheddar.

6. Cover the dish with aluminum foil (or a lid if the baking dish has one) and bake for about 20 minutes or until the cheese melts and the casserole is heated all the way through. Serve immediately. Refrigerate leftovers in an airtight container for up to 1 week. Reheat individual servings for 1 to 2 minutes in the microwave or all at once in a 350°F oven for 15 to 20 minutes.

PER SERVING: Calories: 469;
Total carbs: 2g; **Net carbs: 2g, 1%;**
Total fat: 29g, 56%; Protein: 50g, 43%;
Fiber: 0g; Sugar: 1g

VARIATION 1: Calories: 566;
Total carbs: 6g; **Net carbs: 2g, 5%;**
Total fat: 38g, 60%; Protein: 50g, 35%;
Fiber: 4g; Sugar: 1g

VARIATION 2: Calories: 469;
Total carbs: 2g; **Net carbs: 2g, 1%;**
Total fat: 29g, 56%; Protein: 50g, 43%;
Fiber: 0g; Sugar: 1g

VARIATION 1 **CHICKEN BACON RANCH CASSEROLE WITH AVOCADO:** When the casserole comes out of the oven, top with 1 avocado, diced.

VARIATION 2 **SLOW COOKER CHICKEN BACON RANCH CASSEROLE:** Start with step 2. Combine everything in the slow cooker. Stir to combine and cook for 6 to 8 hours on low heat (or for 2 to 3 hours on high heat).

SPINACH MUSHROOM-STUFFED CHICKEN BREASTS

I don't usually make stuffed chicken breasts because I find them just a little too labor-intensive. But when I do take the time to make them, I'm always impressed by how delicious they are. It just goes to show you what an extra 20 minutes can do for flavor. These chicken breasts are stuffed with sautéed mushrooms and spinach and packed with salty crumbled feta for a dinner that's absolutely delightful. **MAKES 4 SERVINGS**

PREP TIME: 15 minutes
COOK TIME: 30 to 40 minutes

2 tablespoons olive oil, divided

2 garlic cloves

8 ounces mushrooms, sliced

2 cups chopped fresh spinach

4 ounces crumbled feta

Salt

Freshly ground black pepper

4 large boneless skinless chicken breasts

PER SERVING: Calories: 307;
Total carbs: 4g; **Net carbs: 3g, 5%;**
Total fat: 15g, 44%; Protein: 39g, 51%;
Fiber: 1g; Sugar: 3g

VARIATION 1: Calories: 329;
Total carbs: 5g; **Net carbs: 3g, 6%;**
Total fat: 17g, 47%; Protein: 39g, 47%;
Fiber: 2g; Sugar: 2g

VARIATION 2: Calories: 580;
Total carbs: 3g; **Net carbs: 3g, 4%;**
Total fat: 40g, 62%; Protein: 52g, 34%;
Fiber: 0g; Sugar: 1g

1. Preheat the oven to 375°F.

2. In a large nonstick skillet over medium heat, heat 1 tablespoon of olive oil.

3. Add the garlic. Sauté for 1 to 2 minutes until fragrant.

4. Add the mushrooms and cook for 5 to 7 minutes or until browned.

5. Add the spinach and give everything a good stir. Remove the skillet from the heat and transfer the mixture to a medium bowl. Let it cool slightly.

6. Add the feta to the spinach-mushroom mixture and stir to combine. Season with salt and pepper.

7. Make a pocket in each chicken breast: Slice down one side of each breast lengthwise, but don't cut all the way through. Cover the chicken with plastic wrap and gently pound the chicken out to make it a little thinner on each side. Season the chicken with salt and pepper on both sides.

8. Divide the mushroom-spinach-feta filling into 4 portions and stuff each piece of chicken with it. Secure the chicken with a toothpick or two. ➤

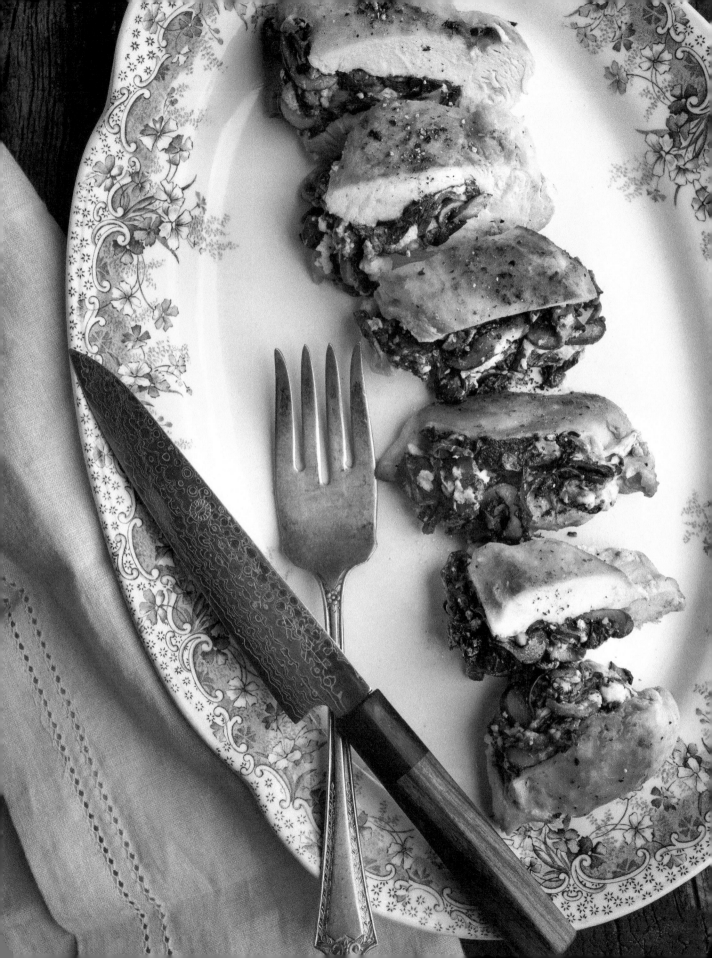

9. Wipe out the nonstick skillet and place it over medium heat. Add the remaining 1 tablespoon of olive oil.

10. Add the chicken breasts to the pan and cook for 4 to 5 minutes per side, just until nicely browned. Transfer the chicken to a baking dish and finish cooking in the oven for 15 to 20 minutes or until the chicken is cooked all the way through and the juices run clear. Refrigerate leftovers in an airtight container for up to 5 days.

VARIATION 1 **SPINACH MUSHROOM–STUFFED CHICKEN BREASTS WITH OLIVES:** Add ½ cup sliced black olives to the spinach-mushroom-feta mixture. Follow the rest of the recipe as written.

VARIATION 2 **PIZZA-STUFFED CHICKEN:** Stuff the chicken with a mixture of 8 ounces chopped pepperoni, 4 ounces shredded mozzarella, and ¼ cup pizza sauce.

MAKE AHEAD: Make the filling and stuff the chicken breasts 1 to 2 days ahead of time. Cover and refrigerate until ready to cook.

EASY MARINATED CHICKEN THIGHS

These easy chicken thighs are great on a busy weeknight. I'm a big fan of chicken thighs rather than breasts for a number of reasons: they're less expensive and they're fattier than breasts, so they're tastier and much harder to overcook. You can throw this recipe together very quickly if you remember to marinate the chicken ahead of time—even overnight, it just gets better and better. These are perfect with some veggies on the side, or topping a plate of salad greens. **MAKES 3 SERVINGS**

PREP TIME: 10 minutes
COOK TIME: 15 minutes
CHILLING TIME: 30 minutes to 2 hours

½ cup olive oil

¼ cup balsamic vinegar

1 teaspoon minced garlic (1 or 2 cloves)

Juice of ½ lemon

½ teaspoon red pepper flakes

1 pound boneless skinless chicken thighs

Salt

Freshly ground black pepper

PER SERVING: Calories: 496; Total carbs: 4g; **Net carbs: 4g, 3%; Total fat: 40g, 73%; Protein: 30g, 24%;** Fiber: 0g; Sugar: 4g

VARIATION 1: Calories: 488; Total carbs: 2g; **Net carbs: 2g, 1%; Total fat: 40g, 74%; Protein: 30g, 25%;** Fiber: 0g; Sugar: 1g

VARIATION 2: Calories: 496; Total carbs: 4g; **Net carbs: 4g, 3%; Total fat: 40g, 73%; Protein: 30g, 24%;** Fiber: 0g; Sugar: 4g

1. In a large container (or in a plastic freezer bag), whisk together the olive oil, vinegar, garlic, lemon juice, and red pepper flakes. Add the chicken and toss well to combine. Season with salt and black pepper. Refrigerate to marinate for at least 30 minutes, and preferably a couple of hours.

2. Cook the chicken on a grill, in a grill pan, large pan, or cast-iron skillet over medium-high heat, for 5 to 7 minutes per side or until browned and cooked through. Serve hot. Refrigerate leftovers in an airtight container for up to 1 week.

VARIATION 1 **SOY LIME CHICKEN BREASTS:** Use the marinade from the Grilled Soy Lime Flank Steak recipe (page 105) instead of the lemon and balsamic marinade for a nice variation in flavor.

VARIATION 2 **BAKED CHICKEN THIGHS:** Instead of cooking these on the stove top, bake them in the oven at 375°F for about 30 minutes or until the juices run clear. Throw them under the broiler for a few minutes at the end to get them nicely browned and crispy.

PERFECT PAIR: Serve with Cheesy Zucchini Gratin (page 219).

UNCLE MARTY'S CHICKEN

My mom always made "Uncle Marty's Chicken" when I was growing up, and not realizing it was a family recipe, I thought it was as familiar to everyone as mac 'n' cheese or pepperoni pizza. My cousin Molly and I were talking about it recently and I laughed so hard when I learned she had felt the same way about it. It's just very thin pieces of chicken breaded and panfried. This is a keto version, so now you, too, can make Uncle Marty's Chicken. **MAKES 4 SERVINGS**

PREP TIME: 10 minutes
COOK TIME: 20 minutes

1½ pounds boneless skinless chicken breasts, halved lengthwise

Salt

Freshly ground black pepper

2 eggs

3 tablespoons heavy (whipping) cream

2 cups almond flour

1 tablespoon dried oregano

1 tablespoon garlic powder

¼ cup olive oil

PER SERVING: Calories: 456;
Total carbs: 6g; **Net carbs: 4g, 5%;**
Total fat: 28g, 56%; Protein: 45g, 39%;
Fiber: 2g; Sugar: 1g

VARIATION 1: Calories: 456;
Total carbs: 6g; **Net carbs: 4g, 5%;**
Total fat: 28g, 56%; Protein: 45g, 39%;
Fiber: 2g; Sugar: 1g

VARIATION 2: Calories: 482;
Total carbs: 6g; **Net carbs: 4g, 5%;**
Total fat: 30g, 56%; Protein: 47g, 39%;
Fiber: 2g; Sugar: 1g

1. Cover the chicken in plastic wrap and use a meat tenderizer or heavy skillet to flatten each piece—pound it pretty vigorously so it is as thin as possible. Season with salt and pepper.

2. In a shallow dish, whisk together the eggs and cream.

3. In another shallow dish, season the almond flour with lots of salt and pepper and stir in the oregano and garlic powder.

4. Place a large skillet over medium-high heat and add the olive oil.

5. Dip each piece of chicken first in the egg wash and then in the almond flour. Coat both sides of the chicken with the flour and carefully transfer the chicken to the hot oil. Cook for about 5 minutes per side or until the almond flour starts to turn golden brown.

6. Remove from the skillet and place on a paper towel-lined platter (you can also transfer the pieces to a baking sheet and keep them warm in a 250°F oven until ready to serve). Refrigerate leftovers in an airtight container for up to 1 week. Reheat in a skillet over medium heat until warmed through.

VARIATION 1 **CHILI LIME UNCLE MARTY'S CHICKEN:** Skip the oregano and season the almond flour with 1 teaspoon ground cayenne pepper and the zest of 1 lime. Serve the chicken with lime wedges.

VARIATION 2 **GARLIC AND HERB UNCLE MARTY'S CHICKEN:** Add 1 tablespoon dried Italian seasoning and ¼ cup grated Parmesan to the almond flour mixture. Follow the rest of the recipe as written.

PERFECT PAIR: Serve with Cheesy Broccoli Casserole (page 184).

7

BEEF

Beef is sometimes a better keto protein option than chicken because the choice of cuts is greater, and you can find some cuts with much higher fat content. I usually have some steaks and a pound or two of ground beef in my refrigerator or freezer at any time—I've found it's the easiest way to throw together a keto-friendly meal without a lot of planning.

Some of my go-to meals are very simple: grilled steaks and a salad, ground beef with some garlic and a side of veggies. The following recipes—from taco salads to kebabs and even stuffed peppers—have a bit more to them but most still take about 30 minutes to prepare.

STEAK SALAD

Whenever I visit my best friend, Tina, in Richmond, Virginia, we have steak salads at the same great place in Carytown. It's one of those traditions that just developed over the years without either of us mentioning it, and now we do it without even thinking. I love it when food does that to friendships.

MAKES 2 SERVINGS

PREP TIME: 10 minutes
COOK TIME: 20 minutes

¾ pound flank steak (or your favorite cut)

1 tablespoon olive oil

Salt

Freshly ground black pepper

1 tablespoon butter

1 head romaine lettuce, chopped

1 small head butter lettuce, chopped

½ cup cherry tomatoes, sliced

½ cup crumbled blue cheese

½ cup Ranch Dressing (page 225)

PER SERVING: Calories: 864; Total carbs: 20g; **Net carbs: 19g, 14%; Total fat: 63g, 65%; Protein: 50g, 23%;** Fiber: 1g; Sugar: 8g

VARIATION 1: Calories: 1096; Total carbs: 29g; **Net carbs: 25g, 12%; Total fat: 83g, 68%; Protein: 52g, 19%;** Fiber: 4g; Sugar: 9g

VARIATION 2: Calories: 966; Total carbs: 21g; **Net carbs: 20g, 10%; Total fat: 65g, 61%; Protein: 70g, 29%;** Fiber: 1g; Sugar: 8g

1. Drizzle the steak with the olive oil and season it with salt and pepper. On a grill or in a cast-iron skillet over medium-high heat, cook the steak for 7 to 8 minutes per side (more or less depending on how you like your steak cooked—this timing will give you medium-rare). Remove the steak from the heat, top with the butter, and let it rest for 10 minutes before slicing.

2. In a large bowl, combine the romaine and butter lettuces, tomatoes, blue cheese, and ranch dressing. Season with a bit more salt and pepper, toss to combine, and divide between two large bowls for serving. Top with sliced steak and enjoy immediately.

VARIATION 1 **STEAK SALAD WITH AVOCADO:** Add ½ avocado, sliced or diced, to each salad for an additional boost of fat.

VARIATION 2 **SURF AND TURF SALAD:** Follow the recipe as written and add 6 grilled shrimp to the salad with the steak.

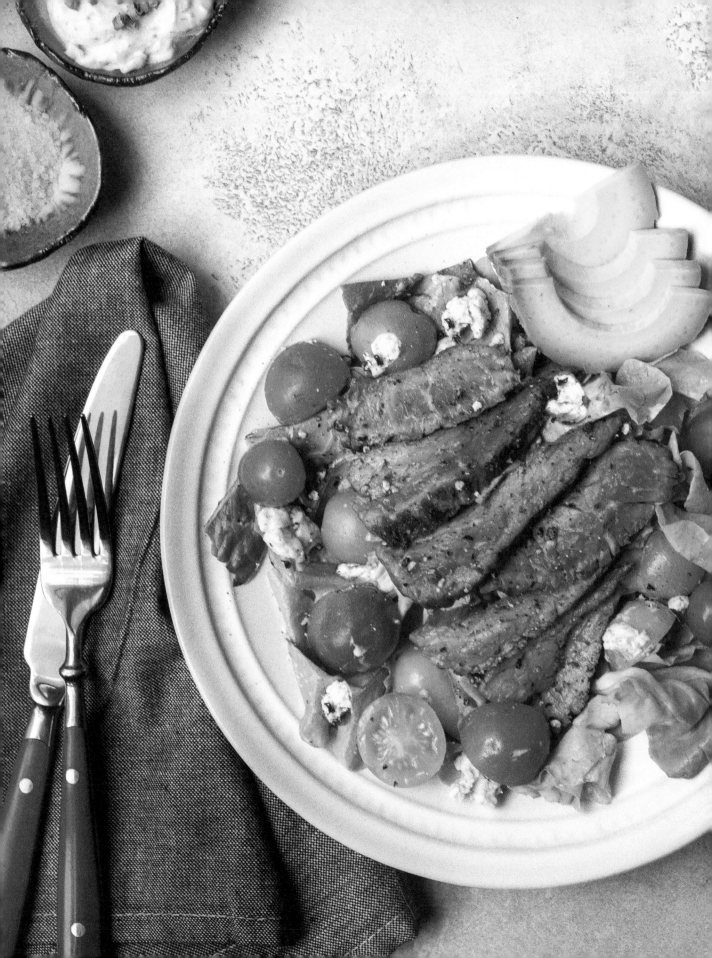

KETO TACO SALAD

I used to make Paleo taco salads a few years ago, and while they're still incredibly tasty, there's something even better about adding shredded cheese and sour cream. This is one of my go-to easy dinners that takes almost no planning to put together. **MAKES 4 SERVINGS**

PREP TIME: 10 minutes
COOK TIME: 15 minutes

1 tablespoon olive oil

½ white onion, diced

1 garlic clove, minced

1 pound ground beef

1 small packet taco seasoning (or 1½ teaspoons chili powder combined with 1½ teaspoons ground cumin)

Salt

Freshly ground black pepper

2 heads romaine lettuce, chopped

½ cup shredded Mexican blend cheese

¼ cup salsa

¼ cup sour cream

1 avocado, quartered and sliced

4 lime wedges

1. In a large saucepan over medium heat, heat the olive oil.

2. Add the onion and garlic. Sauté for 5 to 7 minutes until the onion is softened and translucent.

3. Add the ground beef and cook for 7 to 10 minutes until browned. Season with the taco seasoning, salt, and pepper. Drain and set aside.

4. Assemble the salads in four bowls: Start with lettuce. Top with seasoned ground beef. Sprinkle with cheese and add salsa, sour cream, and sliced avocado, and serve with a lime wedge.

VARIATION 1 **KETO TACO SALAD WITH GUACAMOLE:** Use 3 tablespoons Everyday Guacamole (page 38) instead of sliced avocado on each salad.

VARIATION 2 **KETO TACO SALAD WITH CHICKEN:** Use shredded chicken instead of ground beef—cook 4 boneless skinless chicken breasts in a slow cooker (for 3 to 4 hours on high heat or 6 to 8 hours on low heat) with a jar of your favorite salsa. Shred with two forks and serve on the salads.

PERFECT PAIR: Serve with Cheese Crisps (page 57).

PER SERVING: Calories: 597; Total carbs: 19g; **Net carbs: 15g, 13%;** **Total fat: 41g, 62%; Protein: 38g, 25%;** Fiber: 4g; Sugar: 6g

VARIATION 1: Calories: 619; Total carbs: 20g; **Net carbs: 16g, 12%;** **Total fat: 43g, 63%; Protein: 38g, 25%;** Fiber: 4g; Sugar: 6g

VARIATION 2: Calories: 461; Total carbs: 23g; **Net carbs: 18g, 20%;** **Total fat: 25g, 50%; Protein: 36g, 30%;** Fiber: 5g; Sugar: 8g

STEAK AND MUSHROOM KEBABS

We make kebabs a lot during the summer, especially on weekends; it's so easy to marinate some meat and veggies, skewer them, and take everything out to the grill. There are endless combinations of protein and veggies you can choose from, but these simple steak and mushroom kebabs are my favorite. Try serving them with a side of field greens and some Ranch Dressing (page 225) or a simple vinaigrette. **MAKES 4 SERVINGS**

PREP TIME: 15 minutes
COOK TIME: 15 minutes

1 pound sirloin steak, cut into large cubes

12 ounces white button mushrooms, or baby bella mushrooms

3 tablespoons olive oil

Salt

Freshly ground black pepper

PER SERVING: Calories: 322;
Total carbs: 3g; **Net carbs: 2g, 3%;**
Total fat: 23g, 64%; Protein: 26g, 33%;
Fiber: 1g; Sugar: 1g

VARIATION 1: Calories: 485;
Total carbs: 5g; **Net carbs: 4g, 4%;**
Total fat: 40g, 73%; Protein: 28g, 23%;
Fiber: 1g; Sugar: 2g

VARIATION 2: Calories: 398;
Total carbs: 7g; **Net carbs: 5g, 6%;**
Total fat: 24g, 53%; Protein: 39g, 41%;
Fiber: 2g; Sugar: 3g

1. Preheat the grill to medium-high heat.

2. In a large bowl, combine the cubed steak and mushrooms. Add the olive oil and season with salt and pepper. Toss to combine. Alternate pieces of steak and mushroom on skewers.

3. Grill for 6 to 8 minutes per side. Alternatively, cook the kebabs in a large skillet over medium-high heat. Remove from the heat, slide the steak and mushrooms from the skewers, and serve. Refrigerate leftovers in an airtight container for up to 5 days.

VARIATION 1 **STEAK AND MUSHROOM KEBABS WITH SOY LIME MARINADE:** Use the marinade from the Grilled Soy Lime Flank Steak recipe (page 105) and marinate the steak and mushrooms for 20 to 30 minutes before cooking.

VARIATION 2 **FAJITA KEBABS:** Add ½ pound boneless skinless chicken breasts or thighs, cubed. Season with taco seasoning (or equal parts ground cumin and chili powder), salt, and pepper, and serve with lime wedges.

LOW-CARB CHILI

Chili is a great dish for the fall and winter—it's a little time-intensive to make, but you can make a big batch of it once and feed yourself or your family all week. My brother and I have worked on our recipe a lot, and I tweaked this one to make it lower carb and more keto-friendly: fewer tomatoes, no beans, and don't forget to garnish with a nice scoop of sour cream! This recipe is cozy and comforting and just spicy enough to warm you up on a chilly evening. **MAKES 6 SERVINGS**

PREP TIME: 15 minutes
COOK TIME: 3 hours

2 tablespoons olive oil

1 large onion, diced

3 garlic cloves, minced

1 medium red bell pepper, chopped

1 medium yellow bell pepper, chopped

2 pounds ground beef

1 (6-ounce) can tomato paste

4 cups water

1 tablespoon chili powder

1½ teaspoons red pepper flakes

1 teaspoon ground cumin

1 teaspoon paprika

¾ teaspoon dry mustard

¾ teaspoon ground coriander

½ teaspoon dried oregano

½ teaspoon ground allspice

2 cups beef broth

1½ teaspoons ground cayenne pepper (more or less depending on your heat preference)

½ cup apple cider vinegar

Sliced scallion, green parts only, for garnish

1. In a large saucepan over medium heat, heat the olive oil.

2. Add the onion, garlic, and red and yellow bell peppers. Sauté for about 5 minutes until the vegetables cook down.

3. Add the beef. Cook for 5 to 7 minutes, stirring with a wooden spoon and breaking up the beef until mostly browned.

4. Add the tomato paste and water. Give it a good stir.

5. Stir in the chili powder, red pepper flakes, cumin, paprika, mustard, coriander, oregano, and allspice. Bring the chili to a low boil, reduce the heat to simmer, cover the pan, and cook for at least 2 hours. Periodically check the chili and stir in some broth when it starts getting thick.

6. About 20 minutes before serving, stir in the cayenne and vinegar. Spoon into bowls and top with scallion.

PER SERVING: Calories: 551;
Total carbs: 13g; **Net carbs: 10g, 10%;**
Total fat: 43g, 70%; Protein: 28g, 20%;
Fiber: 3g; Sugar: 7g

VARIATION 1: Calories: 551;
Total carbs: 13g; **Net carbs: 10g, 10%;**
Total fat: 43g, 70%; Protein: 28g, 20%;
Fiber: 3g; Sugar: 7g

VARIATION 2: Calories: 665;
Total carbs: 18g; **Net carbs: 11g, 11%;**
Total fat: 53g, 72%; Protein: 29g, 17%;
Fiber: 7g; Sugar: 7g

VARIATION 1 **SLOW COOKER CHILI:** Follow the recipe through step 3. Transfer everything to a slow cooker. Add the rest of the ingredients and cook for at least 6 hours on low heat.

VARIATION 2 **LOW-CARB CHILI WITH AVOCADO:** Serve each portion of chili with ¼ avocado (and/or a sprinkle of shredded Cheddar) for some extra fat.

PHILLY CHEESESTEAK-STUFFED PEPPERS

These stuffed peppers are a keto take on Philly cheesesteak sandwiches. Instead of being sautéed, the peppers are stuffed with buttery sautéed onions and thinly sliced steak, topped with cheese, and roasted in the oven. I like to make a few at a time and save them for quick lunches throughout the week; they keep pretty well in the refrigerator for up to 3 days and can be reheated in a 350°F oven for 15 to 20 minutes. **MAKES 2 SERVINGS**

PREP TIME: 10 minutes
COOK TIME: 25 minutes

2 tablespoons butter

1 onion, thinly sliced

2 garlic cloves, minced

1 pound steak, such as skirt, flank, or rib eye, thinly sliced

Salt

Freshly ground black pepper

2 green bell peppers, tops removed, peppers seeded and ribbed

2 slices provolone cheese

PER SERVING: Calories: 686; Total carbs: 14g; **Net carbs: 10g, 7%;** **Total fat: 44g, 58%; Protein: 56g, 35%;** Fiber: 4g; Sugar: 7g

VARIATION 1: Calories: 690; Total carbs: 15g; **Net carbs: 11g, 8%;** **Total fat: 45g, 57%; Protein: 57g, 35%;** Fiber: 4g; Sugar: 7g

VARIATION 2: Calories: 1032; Total carbs: 16g; **Net carbs: 12g, 6%;** **Total fat: 89g, 77%; Protein: 42g, 17%;** Fiber: 4g; Sugar: 8g

1. Preheat the oven to 350°F.

2. In a large skillet over medium heat, melt the butter.

3. Add the onion. Sauté for 5 to 7 minutes until the onion is softened and translucent.

4. Add the garlic and give everything a stir.

5. Add the steak and cook for 3 to 5 minutes until browned (the meat doesn't have to be totally cooked—you're going to put it in the oven). Season everything with salt and pepper. Remove from the heat.

6. Put the peppers in a baking dish just large enough to hold them. If necessary, slice a very thin piece from the bottom of each pepper to ensure it stands up straight. Fill each pepper with the steak and onion mixture and top with 1 slice of cheese. Bake for 15 to 20 minutes or until the peppers are fork-tender and the cheese has melted. Serve immediately.

VARIATION 1 **PHILLY CHEESESTEAK-STUFFED PEPPERS WITH MUSHROOMS:** Add ½ cup sliced mushrooms to the onion mixture and cook for 5 to 7 minutes until browned.

VARIATION 2 **CHEESEBURGER-STUFFED PEPPERS:** Instead of steak, use 1 pound ground beef. Add 4 tablespoons Low-Carb Ketchup (page 226) and top with Cheddar instead of provolone.

MAKE AHEAD: Cook the onions and meat and stuff the peppers up to 2 days ahead. Refrigerate until ready to cook. Top with the cheese and bake according to the recipe instructions.

CHEESEBURGER CASSEROLE

When I first developed this recipe, I loved it so much I made it at least once a week—it was so easy to throw together and absolutely delicious. We make burgers without the bun at home a lot, but there's something special about this cheeseburger casserole. It's a little nostalgic in some ways, kind of like a meatloaf, but it's even more comforting and has a ton of extra flavor. I promise you won't even miss the bun when you serve this casserole for dinner. **MAKES 4 SERVINGS**

PREP TIME: 10 minutes
COOK TIME: 35 minutes

1 tablespoon olive oil

¼ white onion, diced

1 pound ground beef

Salt

Freshly ground black pepper

2 eggs

½ cup heavy (whipping) cream

2 tablespoons tomato paste

1 cup shredded Cheddar cheese, divided

PER SERVING: Calories: 667; Total carbs: 4g; **Net carbs: 4g, 2%;** **Total fat: 60g, 81%; Protein: 28g, 17%;** Fiber: 0g; Sugar: 2g

VARIATION 1: Calories: 669; Total carbs: 4g; **Net carbs: 3g, 3%;** **Total fat: 60g, 80%; Protein: 28g, 17%;** Fiber: 1g; Sugar: 2g

VARIATION 2: Calories: 667; Total carbs: 4g; **Net carbs: 4g, 2%;** **Total fat: 60g, 81%; Protein: 28g, 17%;** Fiber: 0g; Sugar: 2g

1. Preheat the oven to 350°F.

2. In a large skillet over medium heat, heat the olive oil.

3. Add the onion and sauté for 5 to 7 minutes until softened and translucent.

4. Add the beef and cook for 5 to 7 minutes until browned, stirring to break up the meat. Season with salt and pepper. Drain and transfer to a 7-by-11-inch baking dish.

5. In a medium bowl, mix together the eggs, cream, tomato paste, and ½ cup of Cheddar. Season with salt and pepper.

6. Pour the cheese mixture over the beef. Gently shake the dish and tap it on the counter to ensure the cheese mixture makes it through to the bottom and sides of the dish. Top with the remaining ½ cup of Cheddar and bake for 25 minutes until the top is set and the cheese has melted.

VARIATION 1 **CHEESEBURGER CASSEROLE WITH GREENS:** Up your greens intake by adding 1 cup chopped fresh spinach or kale to the beef while cooking.

VARIATION 2 **CHEESEBURGER CASSEROLE WITH PEPPER JACK:** Use pepper jack (or whatever your favorite cheese is) instead of the Cheddar for a flavor variation.

MAKE AHEAD: Cook the beef and assemble the casserole the night before, cover, and refrigerate until ready to bake.

THE CLASSIC JUICY LUCY

My husband and I lived in Minneapolis for a year and a half and we loved pretty much everything about it. It took us a few months, but we finally tried a few Juicy Lucys in the area, and they were delicious. What's a Juicy Lucy? It's pretty simple—basically a cheeseburger, but the cheese is inside the burger instead of on top. It seems like a small difference, but the result is a lipsmacking lava flow of cheesy goodness when you bite in. Want one? **MAKES 4 SERVINGS**

PREP TIME: 10 minutes
COOK TIME: 10 minutes

1 pound ground beef

8 ounces Cheddar cheese, shredded or cubed

Salt

Freshly ground black pepper

PER SERVING: Calories: 602;
Total carbs: 1g; **Net carbs: 1g, 1%;**
Total fat: 53g, 78%; Protein: 30g, 21%;
Fiber: 0g; Sugar: 0g

VARIATION 1: Calories: 545;
Total carbs: 1g; **Net carbs: 1g, 0%;**
Total fat: 45g, 74%; Protein: 33g, 26%;
Fiber: 0g; Sugar: 0g

VARIATION 2: Calories: 602;
Total carbs: 1g; **Net carbs: 1g, 1%;**
Total fat: 53g, 78%; Protein: 30g, 21%;
Fiber: 0g; Sugar: 0g

1. Divide the ground beef into 4 equal portions. (This makes 4 quarter-pound burgers—if you want 2 larger ones, just divide the meat in half.) Form each portion into a patty, pressing down on the center to flatten it out a bit.

2. Add ¼ of the Cheddar to the center of each burger and roll the sides of the patty up to cover the cheese, like a big meatball. Smooth the burger out in your hands and gently press down with your palms to re-form it into a patty. Season both sides generously with salt and pepper.

3. In a large skillet, cast-iron pan, or on the grill over medium-high heat, cook the burgers for 7 to 10 minutes per side, depending on how you like them done. This timing will give you medium burgers; cook for a little less time if you prefer yours medium-rare. Remove the burgers from the heat and serve immediately with your favorite keto toppings (lettuce, pickles, sliced onion, Low-Carb Ketchup, page 226, Keto Mayonnaise, page 225).

VARIATION 1 **JUICY LUCY LAMB BURGERS:** For a fancier variation on the classic, use ground lamb instead of beef.

VARIATION 2 **SPICY JUICY LUCY:** Swap in pepper jack cheese for the Cheddar, or add ½ teaspoon red pepper flakes to the burger mix.

PERFECT PAIR: Serve these burgers with a side of Zucchini Fries with Garlic Aioli (page 217).

KETO SLOPPY JOES

Sloppy Joes are one of those things I think I remember from my childhood, but the truth is I never really ate them as a kid. But I love making these keto Sloppy Joes—they are really good on their own, almost like a stew, but you can also serve this over veggies or with a salad. You can make a big batch and have it for lunch throughout the week. **MAKES 2 SERVINGS**

PREP TIME: 5 minutes
COOK TIME: 20 minutes

1 tablespoon olive oil

½ onion, diced

1 garlic clove, minced

1 pound ground beef

¼ cup Low-Carb Ketchup (page 226)

Salt

Freshly ground black pepper

PER SERVING: Calories: 837; Total carbs: 6g; **Net carbs: 5g, 3%; Total fat: 75g, 80%; Protein: 33g, 17%;** Fiber: 1g; Sugar: 5g

VARIATION 1: Calories: 951; Total carbs: 7g; **Net carbs: 6g, 3%; Total fat: 84g, 79%; Protein: 40g, 18%;** Fiber: 1g; Sugar: 5g

VARIATION 2: Calories: 1125; Total carbs: 8g; **Net carbs: 7g, 2%; Total fat: 100g, 80%; Protein: 47g, 18%;** Fiber: 1g; Sugar: 5g

1. In a large skillet over medium-high heat, heat the olive oil.

2. Add the onion and garlic. Sauté for 5 to 7 minutes until the onion is softened and translucent.

3. Add the beef and cook for 5 to 7 minutes until browned, stirring to break up the meat.

4. Stir in the ketchup, and season with salt and pepper. Reduce the heat to low and simmer for 5 to 10 minutes or until slightly thickened. Remove from the heat and serve. Refrigerate leftovers in an airtight container for up to 5 days.

VARIATION 1 **CHEESY KETO SLOPPY JOES:** Add ½ cup shredded Cheddar to the meat mixture before serving. Cook on low for 1 to 2 minutes to melt.

VARIATION 2 **SLOPPY JOE CASSEROLE:** Follow the recipe as written, remove from the heat, and stir in ¼ cup heavy (whipping) cream, 2 beaten eggs, and ½ cup shredded cheese of choice. Transfer to a 7-by-11-inch baking dish. Bake at 350°F for about 20 minutes or until warmed through and the cheese has melted.

KETO MEATLOAF

This is one of those recipes you don't even realize can be made low-carb until you do it. Simply swap in almond flour for the bread crumbs. My mom always made meatloaf for us growing up, and she said we never liked it until we realized it was basically the same recipe she used for her meatballs, which we did like. I always thought that was so funny. **MAKES 8 SERVINGS**

PREP TIME: 10 minutes
COOK TIME: 1 hour

1 pound ground beef

1 pound ground pork

½ onion, minced

2 garlic cloves, minced

½ green bell pepper, minced

2 eggs

¼ cup almond flour

2 tablespoons heavy (whipping) cream

¼ cup Low-Carb Ketchup (page 226), or 1 tablespoon tomato paste, plus more for brushing

Salt

Freshly ground black pepper

1. Preheat the oven to 350°F.

2. In a large bowl, combine the beef, pork, onion, garlic, bell pepper, eggs, almond flour, and cream. Mix everything together well.

3. Add the ketchup, season with salt and pepper, and stir again to combine. Transfer the meat mixture to a 7-by-11-inch baking dish, forming a loaf shape with your hands. Brush with an additional tablespoon or two of ketchup. Bake for about 1 hour or until the meatloaf is cooked all the way through, browned, and has a nice crust on top. Refrigerate leftovers in an airtight container for up to 1 week.

VARIATION 1 **KETO MEATLOAF WITH SPINACH:** Add some extra greens to this meal. Mix in 3 cups chopped fresh spinach with the other ingredients and bake as directed.

VARIATION 2 **KETO MEATLOAF WITH LAMB:** Swap out the beef or pork (or both) for lamb or even venison—really any red meat you like.

PER SERVING: Calories: 381; Total carbs: 2g; **Net carbs: 2g, 2%; Total fat: 32g, 76%; Protein: 20g, 22%;** Fiber: 0g; Sugar: 1g

VARIATION 1: Calories: 383; Total carbs: 3g; **Net carbs: 2g, 3%; Total fat: 32g, 75%; Protein: 20g, 22%;** Fiber: 1g; Sugar: 2g

VARIATION 2: Calories: 391; Total carbs: 2g; **Net carbs: 2g, 2%; Total fat: 33g, 77%; Protein: 20g, 21%;** Fiber: 0g; Sugar: 1g

GRILLED SOY LIME FLANK STEAK

We have this for dinner at least once a week in the summer—we love grilling not only because it's delicious, but also because it cuts down on the dishes we have to do (leaving more time to watch *Game of Thrones*—again). I put this marinade together the first time because it was all we had in the refrigerator, and now we put it on everything—chicken, shrimp, and especially steak. **MAKES 2 SERVINGS**

PREP TIME: 30 minutes
COOK TIME: 15 minutes
Resting time: 20 minutes
to 1 hour

½ cup olive oil

¼ cup gluten-free soy sauce

Juice of ½ lime

1 garlic clove, minced

Salt

Freshly ground black pepper

1 pound flank steak

PER SERVING: Calories: 466;
Total carbs: 2g; **Net carbs: 2g, 1%;**
Total fat: 40g, 76%; Protein: 25g, 23%;
Fiber: 0g; Sugar: 0g

VARIATION 1: Calories: 263;
Total carbs: 2g; **Net carbs: 2g, 2%;**
Total fat: 27g, 92%; Protein: 4g, 6%;
Fiber: 0g; Sugar: 0g

VARIATION 2: Calories: 611;
Total carbs: 18g; **Net carbs: 7g, 10%;**
Total fat: 48g, 70%; Protein: 31g, 20%;
Fiber: 11g; Sugar: 6g

1. In a large container with a lid or in a plastic freezer bag, combine the olive oil, soy sauce, lime juice, garlic, and some salt and pepper. Add the steak and turn it a few times, or cover and shake, to make sure all the meat is covered with marinade. Refrigerate for at least 20 minutes (30 minutes to 1 hour would be best).

2. Remove the steak from the marinade. In a large skillet or on a grill over medium-high heat, cook the steak for 5 to 7 minutes per side. Remove from the heat and let it rest for 5 to 10 minutes before slicing and serving.

VARIATION 1 **GRILLED SOY LIME SHRIMP:** Instead of steak, marinade 1½ pounds shrimp with the tails on. After marinating, skewer and cook over medium-high heat for 2 to 3 minutes per side.

VARIATION 2 **GRILLED SOY LIME FLANK STEAK SALAD WITH GUACAMOLE:** Serve this steak over 2 heads of chopped romaine lettuce with a side of Everyday Guacamole (page 38).

MAKE IT PALEO: Use coconut aminos instead of soy sauce.

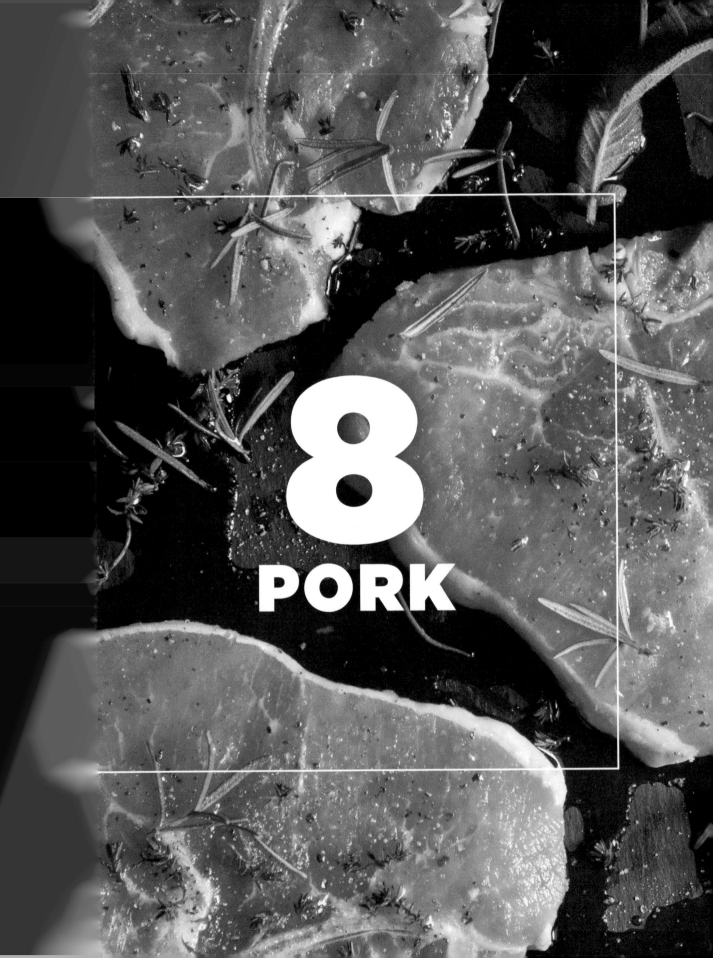

8

PORK

Pork is high in fat, which usually makes most health-conscious dieters stay away from it, but it's probably the best meat for getting and staying in ketosis. In this chapter the recipes range from breakfast to lunch and dinner, with soup and some smaller plates/appetizers thrown in as well. I used to think of pork as a one-trick protein, but you can do all kinds of things with it, and it lends itself well to a wide variety of flavors from Asian to Italian (both of which you'll find in the next few pages).

SAUSAGE BAGELS

This is definitely a "keto hack" if I've ever seen one. Finding work-arounds for bread, bagels, and crackers can be one of the most difficult things about going grain-free or low-carb, especially if up until now you've relied on sandwiches as a go-to lunch or breakfast. As you may have read with the Keto Egg "McMuffins" (page 13), breakfast sandwiches are something I love. A lot. So these sausage bagels have become a staple. **MAKES 2 BAGELS**

PREP TIME: 5 minutes
COOK TIME: 45 minutes

1 pound ground pork

1 teaspoon onion powder

1 teaspoon garlic powder

Salt

Freshly ground black pepper

1 egg

PER SERVING: Calories: 640; Total carbs: 2g; **Net carbs: 2g, 1%;** **Total fat: 51g, 78%; Protein: 42g, 28%;** Fiber: 0g; Sugar: 1g

VARIATION 1: Calories: 884; Total carbs: 3g; **Net carbs: 3g, 1%;** **Total fat: 72g, 73%; Protein: 55g, 26%;** Fiber:0 g; Sugar: 2g

VARIATION 2: Calories: 719; Total carbs: 6g; **Net carbs: 4g, 3%;** **Total fat: 57g, 71%; Protein: 44g, 26%;** Fiber: 2g; Sugar: 1g

1. Preheat the oven to 400°F.

2. In a large bowl, combine the pork, onion powder, and garlic powder. Season with salt and pepper. Stir to combine.

3. In a small bowl, whisk the egg. Add it to the bowl and stir until everything is well incorporated.

4. Divide the pork mixture in half and form two large balls. Use your thumbs to make an indentation in the middle, resembling a bagel. Flatten the balls slightly. Transfer to a small baking dish and bake for 40 to 45 minutes or until the pork is cooked through and meat has browned. Let them cool before slicing and serving.

VARIATION 1 **EGG AND CHEESE ON SAUSAGE BAGELS:** In a large nonstick skillet over medium heat, heat 1 tablespoon olive oil. In a small bowl, whisk 1 egg and pour it into the skillet, letting it spread into a thin layer. Cook for 2 to 3 minutes and flip. Add a slice of your favorite cheese and let it melt. Remove from the heat and serve on the sausage bagel with 1 tablespoon Keto Mayonnaise (page 225).

VARIATION 2 **EVERYTHING SAUSAGE BAGELS:** Before baking, top the sausage bagels with a mix of equal parts sea salt, sesame seeds, and dried onions.

BREAKFAST SAUSAGE AND EGG CASSEROLE

I used to make a breakfast casserole very similar to this one without cheese and with lots of diced sweet potatoes. We have it any time my family or friends gather together for a weekend breakfast. Since going low-carb, I've had to tweak the recipe to make it more keto friendly. This is pretty straightforward—sausage, eggs, and cheese (the best breakfast ingredients, in my opinion). You can make it ahead of time and pop it in the oven to reheat while you brew the coffee. **MAKES 6 SERVINGS**

PREP TIME: 10 minutes
COOK TIME: 1 hour to 1 hour, 25 minutes

3 tablespoons olive oil, divided

¼ onion, chopped

1 garlic clove, minced

10 ounces breakfast sausage

Salt

Freshly ground black pepper

10 eggs

1 cup shredded Cheddar cheese

2 tablespoons sliced scallion, green parts only

PER SERVING: Calories: 406; Total carbs: 2g; **Net carbs: 2g, 2%;** **Total fat: 34g, 75%; Protein: 23g, 23%;** Fiber: 0g; Sugar: 1g

VARIATION 1: Calories: 265; Total carbs: 3g; **Net carbs: 2g, 5%;** **Total fat: 21g, 71%; Protein: 16g, 24%;** Fiber: 1g; Sugar: 2g

VARIATION 2: Calories: 788; Total carbs: 6g; **Net carbs: 4g, 3%;** **Total fat: 72g, 82%; Protein: 29g, 15%;** Fiber: 2g; Sugar: 1g

1. Preheat the oven to 350°F.

2. In a large skillet over medium heat, heat 1½ tablespoons of olive oil.

3. Add the onion and garlic. Sauté for 5 to 7 minutes until the onion is softened and translucent.

4. Add the remaining 1½ tablespoons of olive oil to the skillet along with the sausage. Cook for 5 to 7 minutes or until no pink remains. Season with salt and pepper. Transfer the sausage mixture to a 7-by-11-inch baking dish and arrange in an even layer.

5. In a large bowl, whisk the eggs well, season with salt and pepper, and pour over the sausage layer in the baking dish. Sprinkle with the Cheddar.

6. Bake for 50 minutes to 1 hour, 10 minutes or until the eggs are no longer runny. Serve hot, garnished with a sprinkle of sliced scallion. Refrigerate leftovers in an airtight container for up to 1 week. Reheat in the microwave for about 1 minute or in a 350°F oven for 15 to 20 minutes.

VARIATION 1 **VEGGIE BREAKFAST CASSEROLE:** Skip the sausage and use 10 ounces chopped mushrooms, ½ red bell pepper, diced, and 1 cup chopped fresh spinach. Sauté all the vegetables with the onion and garlic, and mix with the eggs before baking.

VARIATION 2 **BACON AND CHEESE BREAKFAST CASSEROLE WITH AVOCADO:** Use bacon instead of sausage and top this casserole with 1 large sliced avocado. Garnish with chopped fresh cilantro.

ITALIAN SAUSAGE SOUP

Soup is wonderful, especially in the fall and winter. As a kid growing up in Roanoke, Virginia, without a ton of chain restaurants to choose from, Olive Garden was a favorite for soup and salad lunch dates with my friends—it made me feel grown-up. This recipe makes a slightly spicy, comforting, and delicious Italian sausage soup that I serve to my friends now, as a grown-up, with a nice big salad on the side. **MAKES 4 SERVINGS**

PREP TIME: 5 minutes
COOK TIME: 25 minutes

30

1 tablespoon olive oil

½ onion, diced

3 garlic cloves, minced

8 ounces hot Italian sausage, removed from their casings

2 cups chicken broth

1 (14.5-ounce) can diced tomatoes

1 to 2 teaspoons red pepper flakes

1 teaspoon dried oregano

1 teaspoon dried basil

Salt

Freshly ground black pepper

¼ cup freshly grated Parmesan cheese, divided

2 cups chopped fresh spinach

PER SERVING: Calories: 365; Total carbs: 11g; **Net carbs: 9g, 12%; Total fat: 20g, 52%; Protein: 33g, 36%;** Fiber: 2g; Sugar: 4g

VARIATION 1: Calories: 377; Total carbs: 14g; **Net carbs: 12g, 16%; Total fat: 21g, 50%; Protein: 34g, 36%;** Fiber: 2g; Sugar: 4g

VARIATION 2: Calories: 397; Total carbs: 17g; **Net carbs: 13g, 16%; Total fat: 21g, 49%; Protein: 35g, 35%;** Fiber: 4g; Sugar: 7g

1. In a large saucepan over medium heat, heat the olive oil.

2. Add the onion and garlic. Sauté for 5 to 7 minutes until the onion is softened and translucent.

3. Add the sausage to the pan. Cook for about 5 minutes as you crumble it, allowing the meat to brown.

4. Stir in the chicken broth and tomatoes. Bring to a boil and reduce the heat to low.

5. Add the red pepper flakes, oregano, and basil. Season with salt and pepper, and stir in 2 tablespoons of Parmesan. Simmer for 10 minutes and remove from the heat.

6. Stir in the spinach until wilted. Serve sprinkled with the remaining 2 tablespoons of Parmesan.

VARIATION 1 **ITALIAN SAUSAGE SOUP WITH KALE:** Use kale instead of spinach—add it to the pan with the onion and garlic. Follow the rest of the recipe as written.

VARIATION 2 **ITALIAN SAUSAGE SOUP WITH CABBAGE:** Add ½ head cabbage, sliced, to the soup with the onion and garlic. You can do this with the original recipe or variation 1 (cabbage and kale together are delicious).

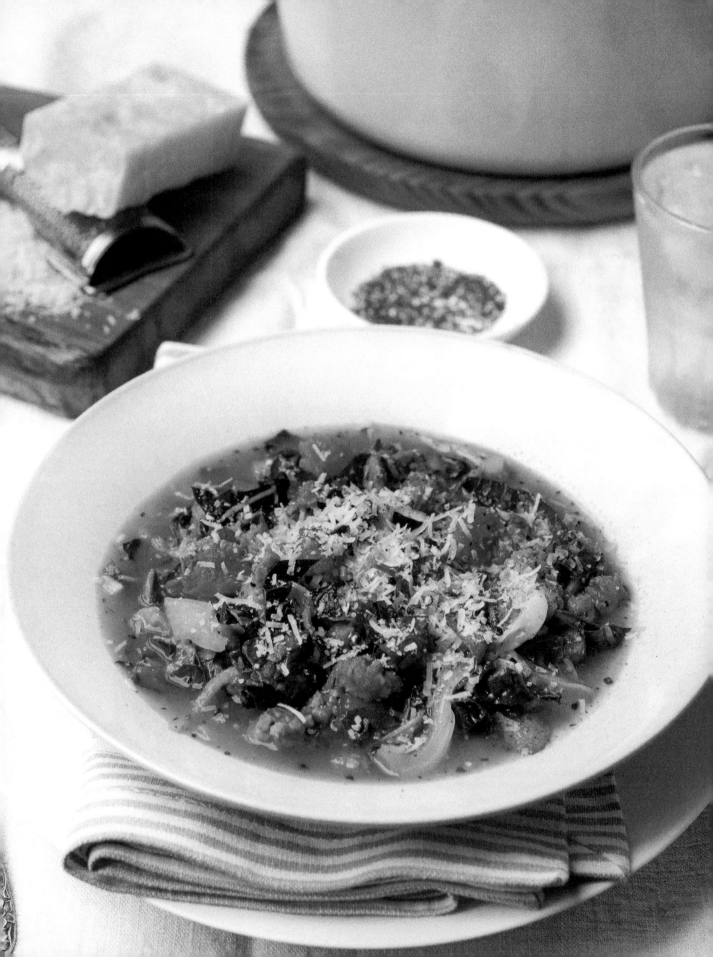

CRISPY PORK LETTUCE WRAPS

Lettuce wraps are the easiest way to make something grain-free and low-carb, and these are great for appetizers or light lunches: crispy pork panfried with sesame and chili oils, a little drizzle of soy sauce, and crisp veggies all nestled in butter lettuce cups with a tangy rice wine vinaigrette. So good. **MAKES 4 SERVINGS**

PREP TIME: 10 minutes
COOK TIME: 10 minutes

2 tablespoons olive oil

2 garlic cloves, minced

¼ cup sesame oil, divided

1 pound pork, sliced thinly

2 to 3 tablespoons gluten-free soy sauce

1 teaspoon chili garlic sauce

2 to 3 tablespoons rice wine vinegar

1 large carrot, julienned

½ large cucumber, julienned

2 tablespoons chopped fresh cilantro

1 small head butter lettuce, or romaine lettuce

PER SERVING: Calories: 340; Total carbs: 8g; **Net carbs: 7g, 9%; Total fat: 24g, 64%; Protein: 23g, 27%;** Fiber: 1g; Sugar: 3g

VARIATION 1: Calories: 399; Total carbs: 8g; **Net carbs: 7g, 8%; Total fat: 27g, 61%; Protein: 31g, 31%;** Fiber: 1g; Sugar: 3g

VARIATION 2: Calories: 448; Total carbs: 12g; **Net carbs: 8g, 10%; Total fat: 34g, 69%; Protein: 24g, 21%;** Fiber: 4g; Sugar: 3g

1. In a large skillet over medium heat, heat the olive oil.

2. Add the garlic and sauté for 1 to 2 minutes until fragrant.

3. Add 2 tablespoons of sesame oil and the pork. Cook for 5 to 6 minutes or until the pork is cooked through and starts to get crispy. Remove from the heat.

4. In a small bowl, whisk the remaining 2 tablespoons of sesame oil, the soy sauce, chili garlic sauce, and vinegar.

5. Add the carrot and cucumber to the dressing and toss to combine.

6. Assemble the lettuce wraps: Layer pork and veggies in lettuce cups and serve with a sprinkle of fresh cilantro.

VARIATION 1 **THAI BEEF LARB LETTUCE WRAPS:** Instead of pork and sesame oil, cook 1 pound ground beef in olive oil or peanut oil with onion and garlic and 1 teaspoon grated fresh ginger. Add a splash of fish sauce and the juice of ½ lime. Serve the lettuce wraps with a sprinkle of fresh mint.

VARIATION 2 **CRISPY PORK LETTUCE WRAPS WITH AVOCADO:** Slice 1 large avocado and add some to each wrap.

EGG ROLL IN A BOWL

This egg roll in a bowl was a game changer for me because it hits all those notes that Asian cuisine usually does, but without breading or sugar or any other excess carbs. I like to buy all the ingredients already chopped, so it comes together really fast for a quick meal. **MAKES 2 GENEROUS SERVINGS**

PREP TIME: 5 minutes
COOK TIME: 15 minutes

1 tablespoon sesame oil

1 pound ground pork

3 garlic cloves, minced

¼ cup gluten-free soy sauce, divided

1 teaspoon red pepper flakes

Salt

Freshly ground black pepper

10 ounces shredded cabbage and carrots (Trader Joe's makes a mix of red and green cabbage with shredded carrots in a 10-ounce bag)

2 teaspoons chili garlic sauce

2 teaspoons rice vinegar

Sliced scallion, green parts only, for topping (optional)

Sesame seeds, for topping (optional)

Hot sauce, for topping (optional)

PER SERVING: Calories: 365; Total carbs: 13g; **Net carbs: 9g, 14%;** **Total fat: 17g, 42%; Protein: 40g, 44%;** Fiber: 4g; Sugar: 5g

VARIATION 1: Calories: 700; Total carbs: 13; **Net carbs: 9g, 8%;** **Total fat: 44g, 57%; Protein: 63g, 36%;** Fiber: 4g; Sugar: 5g

VARIATION 2: Calories: 465; Total carbs:14 g; **Net carbs: 10g, 10%;** **Total fat: 19g, 38%; Protein: 60g, 52%;** Fiber: 4g; Sugar: 5g

1. In a large skillet over medium-high heat, heat the sesame oil.

2. Add the pork. Cook for 5 to 7 minutes, breaking it up with a wooden spoon, until the pork begins to brown and get crispy around the edges.

3. Add the garlic and give it a stir.

4. Add 2 tablespoons of soy sauce and the red pepper flakes. Season with salt (be conservative, you're using soy sauce) and pepper and stir well to combine. Continue to cook until the pork is completely browned, about 5 minutes more.

5. Add the cabbage and carrot mixture to the skillet and reduce the heat to medium. Toss to combine and add the remaining 2 tablespoons of soy sauce and the chili garlic sauce. Cook for 4 to 5 minutes or until the cabbage begins to wilt.

6. Add the vinegar and give everything a good stir. Serve hot, topped with scallion, sesame seeds, and a drizzle of hot sauce (if using).

VARIATION 1 **BEEF EGG ROLL IN A BOWL:** Use 1 pound ground beef instead of pork.

VARIATION 2 **SHRIMP AND PORK EGG ROLL IN A BOWL:** Add 1 cup chopped shrimp to the pork mixture for an even more authentic "egg roll" experience.

ALLERGEN TIP: Swap out the regular soy sauce for tamari, or use coconut aminos if you don't tolerate gluten.

STUFFED PORK ROLL-UPS

These stuffed pork roll-ups are truly delicious and fun—pieces of pork are pounded thin and stuffed with caramelized onions and mushrooms in a luscious cream sauce. They are a little more time-intensive than some recipes in this book, but you can easily make them ahead of time and throw them in the oven once you're ready to serve. To me, the best recipes are the ones that still involve some care and attention to detail, but allow you to spend more time out of the kitchen and with the people you love. **MAKES 4 SERVINGS**

PREP TIME: 15 minutes
COOK TIME: 1 hour

2 tablespoons butter

1 large onion, sliced

2 garlic cloves, minced

10 ounces mushrooms, sliced

Salt

Freshly ground black pepper

4 (4- to 6-ounce) boneless pork chops

½ cup chicken broth

1 teaspoon dried thyme

½ cup freshly grated Parmesan cheese, divided, plus more for garnish

¼ cup heavy (whipping) cream

PER SERVING: Calories: 398;
Total carbs: 8g; **Net carbs: 6g, 8%;**
Total fat: 26g, 60%; Protein: 33g, 32%;
Fiber: 2g; Sugar: 3g

VARIATION 1: Calories: 516;
Total carbs: 8g; **Net carbs: 6g, 6%;**
Total fat: 36g, 63%; Protein: 40g, 31%;
Fiber: 2g; Sugar: 3g

VARIATION 2: Calories: 398;
Total carbs: 9g; **Net carbs: 7g, 9%;**
Total fat: 26g, 60%; Protein: 32g, 31%;
Fiber: 2g; Sugar: 4g

1. Preheat the oven to 350°F.

2. In a large skillet over medium heat, melt the butter.

3. Add the onion and garlic. Sauté for 10 minutes or until the onion begins to caramelize.

4. Add the mushrooms and cook for 8 to 10 minutes or until the mushrooms are golden brown. Season with salt and pepper.

5. While the mushrooms reduce, slice each pork chop in half widthwise, but don't cut all the way through. Open the chop like a book, cover with plastic wrap, and use a meat tenderizer or the back of a heavy pan to pound the meat thinly. Season with salt and pepper and set aside.

6. Once the mushrooms have reduced, stir in the chicken broth and thyme. Bring to a simmer and cook for about 10 minutes or until slightly reduced. Remove from the heat and add ¼ cup of Parmesan and the cream, stirring well to combine.

7. Spoon some mushroom mixture onto the edge of each piece of pork. Add another tablespoon of Parmesan to each and roll up the pork tightly, securing with toothpicks if desired. Transfer to a baking dish large enough to hold them in a single layer, and cover with the remaining mushroom sauce. Bake for 25 to 30 minutes or until the pork is cooked through.

8. Remove the roll-ups from the oven and serve topped with the remaining ¼ cup of Parmesan. Refrigerate leftovers in an airtight container for up to 1 week.

VARIATION 1 **STEAK AND SPINACH ROLL-UPS:** Instead of pork, use thin pieces of steak. Add 2 cups chopped fresh spinach to the mushroom sauce. Follow the rest of the recipe as written.

VARIATION 2 **FETA AND SPINACH PORK ROLL-UPS:** Use feta cheese instead of Parmesan and, instead of putting it in the cream sauce, add it to the pork before rolling. Add 2 cups chopped fresh spinach to the mushroom sauce. Follow the rest of the recipe as written.

MAKE AHEAD: Make the sauce and roll everything up in the baking dish the night before. Cover and refrigerate. Bake about 30 minutes before you're ready to serve.

PEPPERONI PIZZA CASSEROLE

This casserole combines a few of my favorite things: easy meals, keto casseroles, and pizza! I love making casseroles because they're usually too big for just my husband and me so, with leftovers, it's enough for at least two meals. Casseroles are also a delicious way to feed a crowd or simply cut down on your weekly cooking time. This pepperoni pizza casserole will quickly become a family favorite. **MAKES 4 SERVINGS**

PREP TIME: 10 minutes
COOK TIME: 30 minutes

1 tablespoon olive oil

¼ white onion, diced

1 pound pepperoni, roughly chopped

2 teaspoons dried oregano

1 teaspoon red pepper flakes

2 eggs

½ cup heavy (whipping) cream

2 tablespoons tomato paste

1 cup shredded mozzarella cheese, divided

Salt

Freshly ground black pepper

PER SERVING: Calories: 772; Total carbs: 4g; **Net carbs: 3g, 2%; Total fat: 68g, 79%; Protein: 36g, 19%;** Fiber: 1g; Sugar: 2g

VARIATION 1: Calories: 928; Total carbs: 7g; **Net carbs: 5g, 3%; Total fat: 80g, 78%; Protein: 45g, 19%;** Fiber: 2g; Sugar: 3g

VARIATION 2: Calories: 785; Total carbs: 5g; **Net carbs: 3g, 3%; Total fat: 69g, 79%; Protein: 36g, 18%;** Fiber: 2g; Sugar: 2g

1. Preheat the oven to 350°F.

2. In a large skillet over medium heat, heat the olive oil.

3. Add the onion and sauté for 5 to 7 minutes until softened and translucent.

4. Stir in the pepperoni, oregano, and red pepper flakes and remove from the heat.

5. In a medium bowl, whisk the eggs, cream, tomato paste, and ½ cup of mozzarella. Season with salt and pepper and whisk again.

6. Spread the pepperoni and onions in a 7-by-11-inch baking dish. Pour the egg mixture over it. Gently shake the dish and tap it on the counter to ensure the mixture makes it through to the bottom and sides of the dish. Top with the remaining ½ cup of mozzarella. Bake for 25 minutes. Refrigerate leftovers in an airtight container for up to 1 week.

VARIATION 1 **SUPREME PIZZA CASSEROLE:** Add 1 diced green bell pepper, 6 ounces sliced mushrooms, ¼ cup sliced black olives, and 6 ounces cooked sausage to the casserole. Cook according to the instructions.

VARIATION 2 **PEPPERONI PIZZA CASSEROLE WITH OLIVES AND PEPPERONCINI:** Top the casserole with ½ cup sliced black olives. Serve with a side of sliced pepperoncini.

CLASSIC ROAST PORK TENDERLOIN

I made this pork tenderloin one evening when there was nothing else in the refrigerator—I'll occasionally buy a pork tenderloin with no real plans for what to do with it, and most of the time I forget about it and end up throwing it away, which is so frustrating. But with just some salt, pepper, olive oil, and a few spices, we had a delicious dinner that was ready fast. **MAKES 4 SERVINGS**

PREP TIME: 5 minutes
COOK TIME: 25 minutes

   30 DF GF NF

2 tablespoons olive oil

1 (1½-pound) pork tenderloin

1 tablespoon Mrs. Dash Original Seasoning Blend or Trader Joe's 21 Seasoning Salute

Salt

Freshly ground black pepper

PER SERVING: Calories: 323;
Total carbs: 0g; **Net carbs: 0g, 0%;**
Total fat: 20g, 54%; Protein: 35g, 46%;
Fiber: 0g; Sugar: 0g

VARIATION 1: Calories: 323;
Total carbs: 0g; **Net carbs: 0g, 0%;**
Total fat: 20g, 54%; Protein: 35g, 46%;
Fiber: 0g; Sugar: 0g

VARIATION 2: Calories: 384;
Total carbs: 0g; **Net carbs: 0g, 0%;**
Total fat: 26g, 61%; Protein: 35g, 39%;
Fiber: 0g; Sugar: 0g

1. Preheat the oven to 425°F.

2. Drizzle the olive oil over the pork, sprinkle with the seasoning blend, and season with salt and pepper. Place the pork in a baking dish or on a baking sheet. Roast for 20 to 25 minutes or until the internal temperature reaches 145°F.

3. Refrigerate leftovers in an airtight container for up to 1 week.

VARIATION 1 **PAN-SEARED ROAST PORK TENDERLOIN:** If you have a little extra time, sear each side of the tenderloin in a skillet over the hotter side of medium-high heat with 1 tablespoon of olive oil. Just 2 to 3 minutes per side will give it some good color.

VARIATION 2 **SESAME ORANGE PORK TENDERLOIN:** Brush the pork with a mixture of 2 tablespoons sesame oil, 1 tablespoon orange zest, and 1 teaspoon gluten-free soy sauce. Season with salt and pepper and follow the rest of the recipe as written.

PARMESAN-CRUSTED PORK CHOPS

The Parmesan cheese on these pork chops gives them a nice crust without the help of bread crumbs or flour. They're a nice change from the regular, plain ol' grilled meat that I am guilty of making too often when I don't feel too creative, but are just as simple with only a few extra steps. **MAKES 4 SERVINGS**

PREP TIME: 10 minutes
COOK TIME: 15 minutes

 GF

¼ cup grated Parmesan cheese

¼ cup almond flour

1 teaspoon dried parsley

1 teaspoon garlic powder

1 teaspoon onion powder

Salt

Freshly ground black pepper

2 eggs

4 (4- to 6-ounce) boneless pork chops

2 tablespoons olive oil

PER SERVING: Calories: 342; Total carbs: 2g; **Net carbs: 2g, 3%; Total fat: 18g, 48%; Protein: 43g, 49%;** Fiber: 0g; Sugar: 1g

VARIATION 1: Calories: 342; Total carbs: 2g; **Net carbs: 2g, 3%; Total fat: 18g, 48%; Protein: 43g, 49%;** Fiber: 0g; Sugar: 1g

VARIATION 2: Calories: 314; Total carbs: 2g; **Net carbs: 2g, 3%; Total fat: 14g, 40%; Protein: 45g, 57%;** Fiber: 0g; Sugar: 1g

1. In a small shallow dish, combine the Parmesan, almond flour, parsley, garlic powder, onion powder, and some salt and pepper.

2. In another shallow dish, whisk the eggs.

3. Season the pork chops on both sides with salt and pepper. Dip each piece of pork first into the egg and then into the Parmesan-almond flour mixture. Coat the chops thoroughly on both sides.

4. In a large skillet over medium-high heat, heat the olive oil.

5. Add the coated pork chops and cook for 5 to 7 minutes per side or until both sides are browned and the meat is cooked through. Refrigerate leftovers in an airtight container for up to 1 week.

VARIATION 1 **SPICY PARMESAN-CRUSTED PORK CHOPS:** Add 1 teaspoon red pepper flakes to the Parmesan–almond flour mixture.

VARIATION 2 **PARMESAN-CRUSTED CHICKEN BREASTS:** Use boneless skinless chicken breasts instead of pork chops.

PERFECT PAIR: Serve with Warm Spinach Salad (page 206).

FRIED PORK CUTLETS

These fried pork cutlets cook super fast and make a great dinner for busy weeknights. They're really good with a serving of steamed green beans topped with butter and a little salt and pepper—simple and satisfying. These keep pretty well in the refrigerator if you want to make a big batch and reheat them as needed throughout the week, but I think they're best right out of the skillet. **MAKES 4 SERVINGS**

PREP TIME: 10 minutes
COOK TIME: 15 minutes

1½ pounds boneless pork cutlets, or chops, trimmed and pounded to about ¼ inch thick

Salt

Freshly ground black pepper

½ cup almond flour

1 teaspoon garlic powder

1 teaspoon onion powder

1 egg

2 tablespoons heavy (whipping) cream

¼ cup olive oil

PER SERVING: Calories: 372; Total carbs: 2g; **Net carbs: 1g, 2%;** **Total fat: 24g, 58%; Protein: 37g, 40%;** Fiber: 1g; Sugar: 1g

VARIATION 1: Calories: 489; Total carbs: 2g; **Net carbs: 1g, 2%;** **Total fat: 37g, 68%; Protein: 37g, 30%;** Fiber: 1g; Sugar: 1g

VARIATION 2: Calories: 372; Total carbs: 2g; **Net carbs: 1g, 2%;** **Total fat: 24g, 58%; Protein: 37g, 40%;** Fiber: 1g; Sugar: 1g

1. Season the pork cutlets with salt and pepper.

2. In a shallow dish, stir together the almond flour, garlic powder, and onion powder.

3. In another shallow dish, whisk together the egg and cream.

4. Dip each cutlet first into the egg and then into the almond flour mixture. Coat thoroughly on both sides.

5. In a large skillet over medium-high heat, heat the olive oil.

6. Fry the pork cutlets for 4 to 5 minutes per side or until browned and cooked through. Serve immediately.

VARIATION 1 **BUFFALO PORK CUTLETS:** Toss the fried pork cutlets in ¼ cup Frank's RedHot Sauce and ¼ cup melted butter.

VARIATION 2 **RANCH FRIED PORK CUTLETS:** Season the almond flour with ranch seasoning (see the spices from Ranch Dressing, page 225).

9
FISH

Fish seems to be one of those ingredients that people enjoy when they're out, but don't often make at home. I was like that for a long time, too, until I decided to just buy fish and prepare it in my own kitchen—and I was surprised to learn how easy it is. Not only that, but it's also an amazing food to eat regularly. It offers healthy fats and beneficial vitamins and minerals. It's high in protein and low in those healthy fats, which can make it a little tricky for keto, but with the addition of some good oils and dairy products it's something I try to eat two or three times a week.

There are no limits to the delicious seasonings and flavors you can incorporate into your fish dishes. In this chapter you'll find some snacks, lots of dinners, and plenty of recipes that take under 30 minutes to prepare, so you can still make healthy meals even when things get busy.

CREAM CHEESE AND SALMON CUCUMBER BITES

These little bites make the best snack or fancy appetizer for a party. If you're going keto around the holidays, it's helpful to bring a low-carb, high-fat dish to a party so you know you'll have something to eat. (Although what's a party without a big cheese tray? Usually you can find something to nibble on.) This recipe is a tiny bit labor intensive, but there's no cooking and it can be put together in under 30 minutes. **MAKES 6 SERVINGS**

PREP TIME: 15 minutes
COOK TIME: 0 minutes

6 ounces full-fat cream cheese, at room temperature

1 large cucumber, washed, peeled or unpeeled, cut into coins about ½ inch thick (about 12)

6 ounces smoked salmon

Salt

Freshly ground black pepper

PER SERVING: Calories: 126; Total carbs: 3g; **Net carbs: 3g, 6%;** **Total fat: 11g, 70%; Protein: 7g, 24%;** Fiber: 0g; Sugar: 2g

VARIATION 1: Calories: 138; Total carbs: 3g; **Net carbs: 3g, 9%;** **Total fat: 11g, 69%; Protein: 7g, 22%;** Fiber: 0g; Sugar: 2g

VARIATION 2: Calories: 129; Total carbs: 1g; **Net carbs: 1g, 3%;** **Total fat: 11g, 74%; Protein: 7g, 23%;** Fiber: 0g; Sugar: 1g

Spread about ½ ounce of cream cheese onto each cucumber slice. Top each cucumber slice with ½ ounce of smoked salmon. Season with salt and pepper. Serve immediately or refrigerate in an airtight container for up to 2 days.

VARIATION 1 **CREAM CHEESE AND SALMON CUCUMBER BITES WITH RED ONION AND CAPERS:** For an appetizer even more closely resembling a bagel with lox, top each bite with a sprinkle of minced red onion and a few capers.

VARIATION 2 **CREAM CHEESE AND SALMON ZUCCHINI BITES:** Swap out the cucumber slices for zucchini. (I like to slice zucchini a bit thinner than cucumber when I eat it raw.)

POKE SALAD BOWLS

I started eating poke bowls in 2016 when we first moved to California—I think I had at least one a week (often enough that my mom started telling me to lay off because she thought I would get mercury poisoning . . . moms). They're super delicious but I was eating way too much rice, so I started getting them as salads, and I was happy to learn they're just as good on a bed of greens as they are on sushi rice. **MAKES 2 BOWLS**

PREP TIME: 15 minutes
COOK TIME: 0 minutes

¼ cup gluten-free soy sauce

2 tablespoons sesame oil

1 teaspoon chili garlic sauce

2 cups salad greens

¼ pound ahi tuna, diced

¼ pound snow crab leg meat, chopped

½ large cucumber, diced

1 large carrot, julienned or peeled into ribbons

½ avocado, sliced

Sliced scallion, green parts only, for garnish

Sesame seeds, for garnish

3 tablespoons pickled ginger, for garnish (optional)

PER SERVING: Calories: 578; Total carbs: 18g; **Net carbs: 12g, 12%**; **Total fat: 30g, 47%; Protein: 59g, 41%**; Fiber: 6g; Sugar: 5g

VARIATION 1: Calories: 578; Total carbs: 18g; **Net carbs: 12g, 12%**; **Total fat: 30g, 47%; Protein: 59g, 41%**; Fiber: 6g; Sugar: 5g

VARIATION 2: Calories: 1028; Total carbs: 18g; **Net carbs: 12g, 7%**; **Total fat: 80g, 70%; Protein: 59g, 23%**; Fiber: 6g; Sugar: 5g

1. In a large bowl, whisk together the soy sauce, sesame oil, and chili garlic sauce.

2. Add the salad greens and toss to combine. Transfer the greens to two bowls.

3. To the bowl you just tossed the salad in, add the tuna, crabmeat, cucumber, and carrot and toss again. Top the greens with the seafood and veggie mixture.

4. Add the sliced avocado and garnish with scallion, sesame seeds, and pickled ginger (if using). Serve immediately.

VARIATION 1 **SHRIMP AND CRAB SALAD BOWLS:** If you don't want to eat raw fish, swap out the ahi tuna for cooked shrimp (or you can just use crab on its own).

VARIATION 2 **POKE BOWLS WITH CRISPY SHALLOTS:** In a small skillet over medium heat, heat ½ cup vegetable oil. Add 2 or 3 sliced shallots and cook for 5 to 10 minutes, stirring occasionally, until the shallots are browned and crispy. Remove from the skillet and cool slightly before using them to top the salad bowl.

KETO TUNA SALAD

Tuna salad is an easy and inexpensive lunch—I always keep a couple cans of tuna in my pantry, so I'm ready if the refrigerator is looking empty. This version is standard: tuna, some mayo, celery, and a few pickles. You can enjoy it on its own, in a lettuce wrap, or even dip sliced veggies in it. **MAKES 2 SERVINGS**

PREP TIME: 10 minutes
COOK TIME: 0 minutes

2 (5-ounce) cans tuna, drained

¼ cup Keto Mayonnaise (page 225)

½ celery stalk, diced

2 tablespoons finely diced pickles (not sweet)

1 or 2 scallions, green parts only, thinly sliced

Salt

Freshly ground black pepper

In a large bowl, combine the tuna, mayonnaise, celery, pickles, and scallions. Season with salt and pepper. Stir to combine. Serve immediately or refrigerate in an airtight container for up to 4 days.

VARIATION 1 **AVOCADO TUNA SALAD:** Add the juice of ½ lemon and ½ ripe avocado, diced, to the tuna salad instead of the pickles.

VARIATION 2 **SPINACH ARTICHOKE TUNA SALAD:** Add 1 (14-ounce) can artichoke hearts, chopped, and ½ cup chopped fresh spinach to the tuna salad. You may want to increase the mayonnaise to ½ cup.

PERFECT PAIR: Serve this tuna salad over Warm Spinach Salad (page 206) for a more complete meal.

PER SERVING: Calories: 302; Total carbs: 5g; **Net carbs: 4g, 6%;** **Total fat: 16g, 47%; Protein: 34g, 47%;** Fiber: 1g; Sugar: 2g

VARIATION 1: Calories: 391; Total carbs: 11g; **Net carbs: 6g, 10%;** **Total fat: 23g, 52%; Protein: 35g, 38%;** Fiber: 5g; Sugar: 3g

VARIATION 2: Calories: 550; Total carbs: 26g; **Net carbs: 18g, 10%;** **Total fat: 37g, 59%; Protein: 40g, 31%;** Fiber: 8g; Sugar: 1g

CURRIED FISH STEW

I don't make fish stews or soups very often, but when I do they usually have some Italian flavors to them. This one is different because it is seasoned with curry powder and gets its creamy richness from coconut milk. I like making it super spicy but you can control the heat level according to your taste preferences. Normally a stew like this might have potatoes in it, but I use cauliflower to give it some texture while keeping the carb count under control. **MAKES 6 SERVINGS**

PREP TIME: 10 minutes
COOK TIME: 20 minutes

1 tablespoon olive oil

1 medium onion, chopped

3 garlic cloves, minced

1 tablespoon tomato paste

2 tablespoons curry powder

1 head cauliflower, chopped

2 cups fish broth, or vegetable broth

1½ pounds firm whitefish (cod or halibut), cubed

1 teaspoon ground cayenne pepper (more or less depending on your taste)

Salt

Freshly ground black pepper

1 (13.5-ounce) can full-fat coconut milk

1. In a large saucepan over medium heat, heat the olive oil.

2. Add the onion and garlic. Sauté for 5 to 7 minutes until the onion is softened and translucent.

3. Stir in the tomato paste, curry powder, and cauliflower. Cook for 1 to 2 minutes.

4. While stirring, slowly add the broth. Bring to a simmer and add the fish. Cook for 10 to 15 minutes or until the fish is opaque. Season with the cayenne and some salt and pepper.

5. Stir in the coconut milk. Simmer on low until ready to serve. Refrigerate leftovers in an airtight container for up to 4 days.

VARIATION 1 **CURRIED SEAFOOD STEW:** Use just ½ pound fish and add ½ pound shrimp and another ½ pound shellfish (or a second type of fish) for more variety.

VARIATION 2 **FISH STEW:** Skip the curry and season the stew with 1 teaspoon dried oregano and 1 teaspoon dried thyme. Add a few dashes of your favorite hot sauce and follow the rest of the recipe as written.

PERFECT PAIR: Serve the stew over a bowl of Cauliflower Rice (page 178). You can skip the cauliflower in the original recipe if you want.

PER SERVING: Calories: 373; Total carbs: 13g; **Net carbs: 8g, 14%; Total fat: 21g, 51%; Protein: 33g, 35%;** Fiber: 5g; Sugar: 6g

VARIATION 1: Calories: 369; Total carbs: 13g; **Net carbs: 8g, 14%; Total fat: 21g, 51%; Protein: 32g, 35%;** Fiber: 5g; Sugar: 6g

VARIATION 2: Calories: 373; Total carbs: 13g; **Net carbs: 8g, 14%; Total fat: 21g, 51%; Protein: 33g, 35%;** Fiber: 5g; Sugar: 6g

KETO FISH CAKES WITH GARLIC AIOLI

These fish cakes are a great way to use any whitefish you might have sitting around in your fridge. I know sometimes I buy fish with the best intentions, but then can't figure out what to do with it other than just quickly cooking it in some butter or olive oil, which is delicious but can get kind of boring after a while. I love this recipe because it produces something completely new and different, and the mustard with lemon and spices make for an incredibly delicious way to enjoy what might otherwise be bland fish. **MAKES 4 SERVINGS**

PREP TIME: 15 minutes
COOK TIME: 45 minutes

FOR THE AIOLI

1 head garlic, top sliced off to expose the cloves

½ cup Keto Mayonnaise (page 225)

1½ teaspoons olive oil

TO MAKE THE AIOLI

1. Preheat the oven to 400°F.

2. Place the garlic on a piece of aluminum foil big enough to wrap it in. Coat the garlic with olive oil and wrap it in the foil. Bake for 30 to 35 minutes or until softened. Let cool completely.

3. Pop the roasted garlic cloves out of their skins and into a blender. Add the mayonnaise and blend until smooth.

2 (6-ounce) whitefish fillets such as halibut, chopped into a fine mince

¼ cup Keto Mayonnaise (page 225)

2 tablespoons almond flour

2 tablespoons Dijon mustard

1 large shallot, minced

Zest of 1 lemon

Juice of ½ lemon

¼ cup minced fresh parsley leaves

1 egg, slightly beaten

1 teaspoon paprika

Salt

Freshly ground black pepper

2 tablespoons olive oil

PER SERVING: Calories: 318; Total carbs: 9g; **Net carbs: 6g, 12%;** **Total fat: 22g, 62%; Protein: 21g, 26%;** Fiber: 3g; Sugar: 0g

VARIATION 1: Calories: 292; Total carbs: 9g; **Net carbs: 6g, 12%;** **Total fat: 20g, 62%; Protein: 19g, 26%;** Fiber: 3g; Sugar: 0g

VARIATION 2: Calories: 342; Total carbs: 9g; **Net carbs: 6g, 10%;** **Total fat: 22g, 58%; Protein: 27g, 32%;** Fiber: 3g; Sugar: 0g

TO MAKE THE FISH CAKES

1. While the garlic cools, in a large bowl, combine the fish, mayonnaise, almond flour, mustard, shallot, lemon zest and juice, parsley, egg, and paprika. Season with salt and pepper. Mix well to combine. Shape the fish mixture into 4 large cakes or 8 smaller ones (easier to turn when cooking).

2. In a large nonstick skillet over medium-high heat, heat the olive oil. When hot, add the fish cakes. Cook for 4 to 5 minutes until browned. Gently flip each cake, reshaping as needed. Cook for 4 to 5 minutes more until browned. Serve with the garlic aioli. Refrigerate leftovers in an airtight container for up to 4 days.

VARIATION 1 **CRAB CAKES:** Use canned crabmeat instead of fish.

VARIATION 2 **SALMON CAKES:** Use canned or baked salmon instead of whitefish.

LOW-CARB FRIED FISH FILLETS WITH TARTAR SAUCE

Is there anything better than fried seafood with cool, creamy tartar sauce? There's something about it that just brings my mind to the beach every time—probably because I really only have it when I'm on vacation somewhere. These low-carb fish fillets are quickly battered and fried in oil, then served with an easy homemade tartar sauce so you can enjoy them anytime—not just by the ocean with a drink in your hand! **MAKES 4 SERVINGS**

PREP TIME: 15 minutes
COOK TIME: 10 minutes

FOR THE FISH FILLETS

½ cup almond flour

1 teaspoon garlic powder

1 teaspoon paprika

Salt

Freshly ground black pepper

1 egg

2 tablespoons heavy (whipping) cream

4 (4- to 6-ounce) whitefish pieces, such as cod or tilapia

¼ cup olive oil

Lemon wedges, for serving

TO MAKE THE FISH FILLETS

1. In a shallow dish, combine the almond flour, garlic powder, paprika, and some salt and pepper.

2. In another shallow dish, whisk together the egg and cream.

3. Pat the fish dry with paper towels and season with salt and pepper.

4. In a large skillet over medium-high heat, heat the olive oil.

5. Dip each fish fillet first in the egg and then in the almond flour mixture. Coat both sides well. Place each piece of fish into the hot oil and cook for 2 to 3 minutes per side or until the almond flour is brown and crispy. Serve with the tartar sauce and lemon wedges.

FOR THE TARTAR SAUCE

1 cup Keto Mayonnaise
(page 225)

1 tablespoon pickle relish
(not sweet)

1 tablespoon minced onion

Juice of ½ lemon

Salt

Freshly ground black pepper

PER SERVING: Calories: 572;
Total carbs: 10g; **Net carbs: 9g, 7%;**
Total fat: 40g, 63%; Protein: 43g, 30%;
Fiber: 1g; Sugar: 1g

VARIATION 1: Calories: 499;
Total carbs: 10g; **Net carbs: 9g, 8%;**
Total fat: 39g, 70%; Protein: 27g, 22%;
Fiber: 1g; Sugar: 1g

VARIATION 2: Calories: 229;
Total carbs: 9g; **Net carbs: 7g, 16%;**
Total fat: 13g, 51%; Protein: 19g, 33%;
Fiber: 2g; Sugar: 5g

TO MAKE THE TARTAR SAUCE

In a medium bowl, stir together the mayonnaise, relish, onion, and lemon juice. Season with salt and pepper. Stir again until mixed thoroughly. Refrigerate until serving.

VARIATION 1 **FRIED SHRIMP WITH TARTAR SAUCE:** Use 1 pound shrimp, deveined, instead of fish (I use shrimp with the tails on).

VARIATION 2 **FRIED FISH (OR SHRIMP) WITH KETO COCKTAIL SAUCE:** Instead of tartar sauce, mix 1 cup Low-Carb Ketchup (page 226) with 1 tablespoon prepared horseradish, a squeeze of fresh lemon juice, and a splash of Worcestershire sauce. Season with salt and pepper.

SALMON ROMESCO

This romesco sauce is delicious and versatile and definitely not just for salmon! It's also wonderful on chicken and even as a dip for veggies. That said, it's especially delicious on salmon. I like to make a double batch and serve half of it on the fish and freeze the other half for later. **MAKES 4 SERVINGS**

PREP TIME: 10 minutes
COOK TIME: 30 minutes

 DF **GF**

½ cup almonds

4 garlic cloves, peeled

1 tomato

4 (6-ounce) salmon fillets

2 red bell peppers

¼ cup olive oil

2 tablespoons white wine vinegar

1 tablespoon smoked paprika

1 teaspoon ground cayenne pepper

Salt

Freshly ground black pepper

PER SERVING: Calories: 513; Total carbs: 8g; **Net carbs: 4g, 6%;** **Total fat: 37g, 65%; Protein: 37g, 29%;** Fiber: 4g; Sugar: 3g

VARIATION 1: Calories: 402; Total carbs: 8g; **Net carbs: 4g, 8%;** **Total fat: 22g, 50%; Protein: 43g, 42%;** Fiber: 4g; Sugar: 3g

VARIATION 2: Calories: 513; Total carbs: 8g; **Net carbs: 4g, 6%;** **Total fat: 37g, 65%; Protein: 37g, 29%;** Fiber: 4g; Sugar: 3g

1. Preheat the oven to 375°F.

2. On a large baking sheet, spread out the almonds and add the garlic and tomato. Roast for 10 minutes or until the almonds are fragrant and just starting to brown. Remove the almonds and continue roasting the garlic and tomato for 15 to 20 minutes more until the garlic is browned and the tomato has softened.

3. While the almonds, garlic, and tomato roast, on a separate baking sheet, bake the salmon for 30 to 35 minutes or until the flesh is opaque and flakes easily with a fork.

4. Meanwhile, roast the red peppers for 3 to 5 minutes over an open flame or on a hot (medium high) grill until the skins are blackened. Cover with plastic wrap and let sweat until cool enough to handle. Peel off the blackened skin and remove the seeds.

5. In a food processor, combine the almonds, garlic, tomato, bell peppers, olive oil, vinegar, paprika, cayenne, and some salt and pepper. Purée until smooth. Serve over the salmon and enjoy immediately.

VARIATION 1 **CHICKEN ROMESCO:** Serve this sauce over baked boneless, skinless chicken breasts.

VARIATION 2 **POACHED SALMON IN ROMESCO:** Instead of baking the salmon, cook it in a skillet with romesco sauce for 5 to 10 minutes per side or until the fish is opaque and the flesh flakes easily with a fork. Serve topped with more sauce.

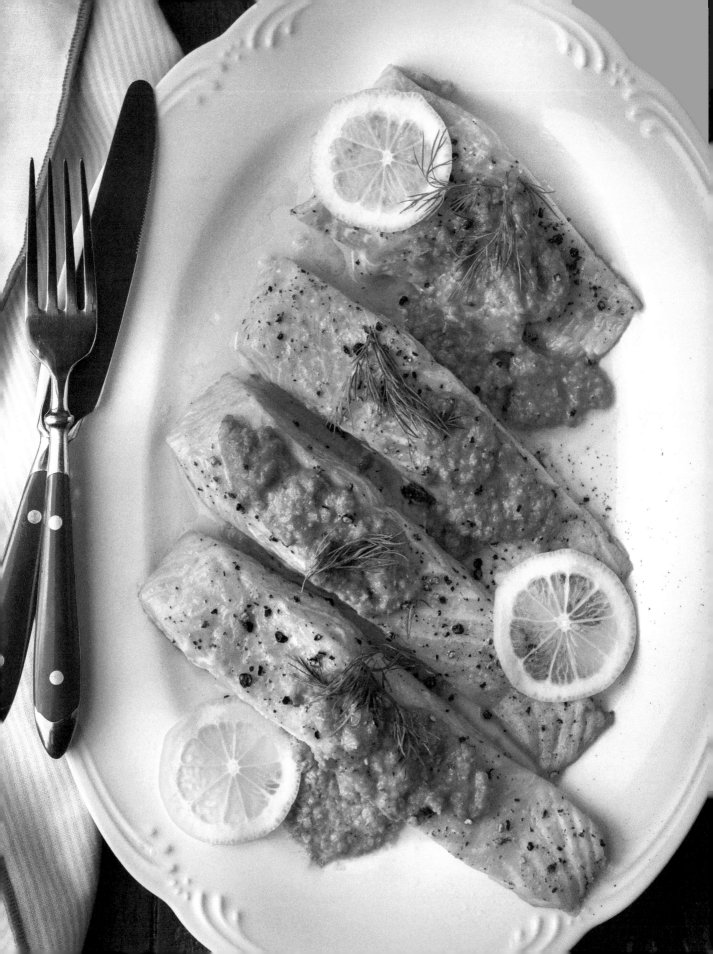

BASIL ALFREDO SEA BASS

This recipe is for a simple baked fish, but the sauce is what makes it really special. It's a combination of two sauces—pesto and Alfredo—that make a great team. **MAKES 4 SERVINGS**

PREP TIME: 15 minutes
COOK TIME: 30 minutes

FOR THE SEA BASS

4 (6-ounce) sea bass pieces

2 tablespoons olive oil

FOR THE PESTO

1 cup tightly packed fresh basil leaves

¼ cup grated Parmesan cheese

3 tablespoons pine nuts, or walnuts

1 tablespoon water

½ teaspoon salt

Freshly ground black pepper

3 tablespoons olive oil

PER SERVING: Calories: 768;
Total carbs: 4g; **Net carbs: 4g, 2%;**
Total fat: 64g, 73%; Protein: 45g, 25%;
Fiber: 0g; Sugar: 1g

VARIATION 1: Calories: 776;
Total carbs: 6g; **Net carbs: 5g, 2%;**
Total fat: 64g, 73%; Protein: 45g, 25%;
Fiber: 1g; Sugar: 1g

VARIATION 2: Calories: 907;
Total carbs: 4g; **Net carbs: 4g, 2%;**
Total fat: 78g, 76%; Protein: 47g, 22%;
Fiber: 0g; Sugar: 1g

TO MAKE THE SEA BASS

1. Preheat the oven to 375°F.

2. Rub the sea bass with the olive oil and place it in a baking dish or on a rimmed baking sheet. Bake for 20 to 25 minutes or until the fish is completely opaque and the flesh flakes easily with a fork.

TO MAKE THE PESTO

1. In a blender or food processor (I prefer a blender because I like this very finely chopped/blended), combine the basil, Parmesan, pine nuts, water, and salt. Season with pepper.

2. With the blender running, stream the olive oil in. Set aside.

FOR THE ALFREDO SAUCE

2 tablespoons butter

1 tablespoon olive oil

1 garlic clove, minced

1 cup heavy (whipping) cream

¾ cup Parmesan cheese

Salt

Freshly ground black pepper

TO MAKE THE ALFREDO SAUCE

1. In a small saucepan over medium heat, melt the butter and olive oil together.

2. Stir in the garlic and cream. Bring to a low simmer and cook for 5 to 7 minutes until thickened.

3. Slowly add the Parmesan, stirring well to mix as it melts. Continue to stir until smooth. Season with salt and pepper. Set aside.

4. In a small bowl, stir together ½ cup of pesto and ½ cup of Alfredo sauce. Spoon over the fish before serving. Refrigerate leftovers in an airtight container for up to 4 days.

VARIATION 1 **KALE PESTO ALFREDO SEA BASS:** Add a handful of kale to the pesto to pack more veggies into this dinner.

VARIATION 2 **PESTO ALFREDO SALMON:** Pour the sauce over baked salmon (see cooking instructions for the fish in Oven-Baked Dijon Salmon, page 134).

MAKE IT PALEO: Swap the heavy cream for coconut cream and skip the Parmesan in the pesto for a dairy-free, Paleo version.

OVEN-BAKED DIJON SALMON

This oven-baked salmon is a favorite because it's almost like a one-pot meal but even faster! Salmon is really great when it's not overdone, so it just needs 10 minutes or so in a hot oven to cook to perfection. Brushed with a little Dijon and served with a side of veggies, you've got an easy and healthy meal in no time at all. **MAKES 4 SERVINGS**

PREP TIME: 5 minutes
COOK TIME: 10 minutes

4 (6-ounce) salmon fillets

2 tablespoons olive oil

Salt

Freshly ground black pepper

¼ cup grainy Dijon mustard

PER SERVING: Calories: 370; Total carbs: 1g; **Net carbs: 0g, 1%;** **Total fat: 25g, 60%; Protein: 34g, 39%;** Fiber: 1g; Sugar: 0g

VARIATION 1: Calories: 386; Total carbs: 5g; **Net carbs: 4g, 4%;** **Total fat: 25g, 58%; Protein: 34g, 38%;** Fiber: 1g; Sugar: 4g

VARIATION 2: Calories: 374; Total carbs: 1g; **Net carbs: 0g, 1%;** **Total fat: 25g, 60%; Protein: 34g, 39%;** Fiber: 1g; Sugar: 0g

1. Preheat the oven to 450°F.

2. Drizzle the fillets with the olive oil and season with salt and pepper. Brush the mustard over each piece of fish and place on a baking sheet. Bake for 10 to 12 minutes or until the salmon is opaque and flakes easily with a fork. (Cook a few minutes longer if you prefer it cooked more than medium.)

VARIATION 1 **HONEY MUSTARD OVEN-BAKED SALMON:** If you have room in your macros for a few more carbs, mix 1 tablespoon honey into the mustard before brushing it onto the fish.

VARIATION 2 **CURRY TURMERIC MUSTARD OVEN-BAKED SALMON:** Add 1 teaspoon ground turmeric and 1 teaspoon curry powder to the mustard before brushing it onto the fish.

PERFECT PAIR: Serve with Warm Spinach Salad (page 206), Zucchini Fries with Garlic Aioli (page 217), or Roasted Lemon Garlic Broccoli (page 188)

SOLE MEUNIÈRE

The first time I learned about sole meunière was through Julia Child; I love the story of her first time in France, eating this dish and being so amazed by the beautiful, tasty simplicity of it. This dish really is delicious, and it's surprisingly easy to make—only a few ingredients are needed, and the fish is nice and thin so it cooks really quickly in the butter. It is basically poached in the pan, which gives it the most luxurious texture. **MAKES 2 SERVINGS**

PREP TIME: 5 minutes
COOK TIME: 10 minutes

½ cup almond flour

4 (6-ounce) sole fillets

Salt

Freshly ground black pepper

6 tablespoons butter, divided

Juice of ½ lemon

2 tablespoons minced fresh parsley leaves

4 lemon wedges (from the other half of the lemon), for serving

PER SERVING: Calories: 624; Total carbs: 2g; **Net carbs: 2g, 1%;** **Total fat: 40g, 55%; Protein: 65g, 44%;** Fiber: 0g; Sugar: 0g

VARIATION 1: Calories: 648; Total carbs: 2g; **Net carbs: 2g, 2%;** **Total fat: 42g, 56%; Protein: 69g, 42%;** Fiber: 0g; Sugar: 0g

VARIATION 2: Calories: 624; Total carbs: 2g; **Net carbs: 2g, 1%;** **Total fat: 40g, 55%; Protein: 65g, 44%;** Fiber: 0g; Sugar: 0g

1. Put the almond flour into a shallow dish.

2. Pat the fish dry with a paper towel and coat each side with almond flour. Season with salt and pepper.

3. In a large skillet over medium heat, melt 3 tablespoons of butter.

4. Add the fish to the skillet and cook for 2 to 3 minutes per side or until the fish is completely opaque. Transfer the fish to a serving platter.

5. Return the skillet to the heat and add the remaining 3 tablespoons of butter and the lemon juice. When melted, pour it over the fish, garnish with the parsley, and serve with the lemon wedges. Refrigerate leftovers in an airtight container for up to 4 days.

VARIATION 1 **TILAPIA MEUNIÈRE:** Use tilapia fillets if you have trouble finding sole, or you just prefer it.

VARIATION 2 **OVEN-BAKED SOLE MEUNIÈRE:** Bake the dredged sole fillets at 350°F for 5 to 10 minutes or until the flesh is completely opaque. Make the sauce as directed and pour it over the cooked fish.

10
SHELLFISH

Shrimp, clams, crab, lobster—if it has a shell on it, you can bet I'm going to eat it and love it. The majority of shellfish you'll find in this chapter are shrimp, crab, and clams, but you can easily swap clams for mussels if you prefer them. I also love raw oysters when I'm out and about but don't generally buy them to prepare at home, so all these recipes are cooked. There are salads, several main courses, and quite a few appetizers, so you'll always have ideas for something fun to do with shellfish when you find yourself at the seafood counter at the store.

SHRIMP ALFREDO

Is there anything better than Alfredo sauce? Garlic, butter, cream, and a little Parmesan for a nice bite. Add succulent sautéed shrimp and you've got a delicious main course just waiting for some veggies on the side to make a really enjoyable ketogenic dinner. **MAKES 2 SERVINGS**

PREP TIME: 10 minutes
COOK TIME: 10 minutes

2 tablespoons butter

2 tablespoons olive oil, divided

1 garlic clove, minced

1 cup heavy (whipping) cream

¾ cup grated Parmesan cheese

Salt

Freshly ground black pepper

1 pound shrimp, shells and tails removed, deveined

PER SERVING: Calories: 1034; Total carbs: 7g; **Net carbs: 7g, 3%; Total fat: 84g, 71%; Protein: 63g, 26%;** Fiber: 0g; Sugar: 1g

VARIATION 1: Calories: 1037; Total carbs: 8g; **Net carbs: 8g, 3%; Total fat: 84g, 71%; Protein: 63g, 26%;** Fiber: 0g; Sugar: 1g

VARIATION 2: Calories: 1043; Total carbs: 5g; **Net carbs: 5g, 2%; Total fat: 82g, 70%; Protein: 69g, 28%;** Fiber: 0g; Sugar: 1g

1. In a small saucepan over medium-low heat, melt together the butter and 1 tablespoon of olive oil.

2. Stir in the garlic and cream. Bring to a low simmer and cook for 5 to 7 minutes until thickened.

3. Slowly add the Parmesan, stirring well to mix as it melts. Continue to stir until smooth. Season with salt and pepper. Set aside.

4. In a skillet over medium heat, heat the remaining 1 tablespoon of olive oil.

5. Add the shrimp and sauté for about 3 minutes per side or until they turn pink. Remove from the heat and toss with the Alfredo sauce. Serve immediately. Refrigerate leftovers in an airtight container for up to 5 days.

VARIATION 1 **SHRIMP ZUCCHINI-FETTUCCINI ALFREDO:** Use a spiralizer to make veggie noodles from 2 large zucchini. Sauté the zucchini for about 3 minutes over medium heat in the same pan you used for the shrimp. Toss in the Alfredo sauce. Serve with the shrimp on top and another sprinkle of Parmesan.

VARIATION 2 **CHICKEN ALFREDO:** Instead of shrimp, use cubed boneless skinless chicken breast. Sauté for 7 for 10 minutes over medium heat until browned and cooked all the way through.

KETO SHRIMP COCKTAIL

I love shrimp cocktail because it's so easy and I know exactly what I'm getting, especially when I'm trying to eat clean or low-carb. Unfortunately, cocktail sauce (anything with ketchup, really) is usually packed with sugar, so it's not exactly keto friendly. This shrimp cocktail is made with low-carb ketchup, so enjoy it guilt-free the next time you find yourself craving a fancy shrimp cocktail! **MAKES 4 SERVINGS**

PREP TIME: 5 minutes
COOK TIME: 0 minutes

1 cup Low-Carb Ketchup (page 226)

1 tablespoon prepared horseradish

Juice of ½ lemon

1 teaspoon Worcestershire sauce

Salt

Freshly ground black pepper

1 pound jumbo shrimp, tails on, cooked

PER SERVING: Calories: 170; Total carbs: 12g; **Net carbs: 10g, 27%; Total fat: 2g, 12%; Protein: 25g, 61%;** Fiber: 2g; Sugar: 7g

VARIATION 1: Calories: 206; Total carbs: 14g; **Net carbs: 12g, 26%; Total fat: 5g, 21%; Protein: 26g, 53%;** Fiber: 2g; Sugar: 8g

VARIATION 2: Calories: 175; Total carbs: 12g; **Net carbs: 10g, 26%; Total fat: 2g, 9%; Protein: 28g, 65%;** Fiber: 2g; Sugar: 7g

In a small bowl, stir together the ketchup, horseradish, lemon juice, Worcestershire sauce, and some salt and pepper. Spoon the cocktail sauce into a smaller dish in the middle of a platter and surround it with the shrimp. Serve immediately or refrigerate for up to 2 days.

VARIATION 1 **CREAMY SHRIMP COCKTAIL:** Add 2 tablespoons Keto Mayonnaise (page 225) to the cocktail sauce to make a creamier version.

VARIATION 2 **CRAB COCKTAIL:** Instead of shrimp, switch it up for jumbo lump crabmeat.

MAKE AHEAD: Make the cocktail sauce a few days ahead of time and prepare the shrimp a few minutes before serving.

CRAB LOUIE SALAD

During the summer my mom makes Louie dressing for salads topped with seafood—I had no idea it is just mayo and ketchup with some spices. I loved it and was so impressed she could whip up something so good with just a few ingredients. **MAKES 2 SERVINGS**

PREP TIME: 10 minutes
COOK TIME: 0 minutes

1 small head butter lettuce, washed and stemmed

2 hardboiled eggs, peeled and halved

2 radishes, thinly sliced

1 medium avocado, sliced

1 medium Roma tomato, quartered

½ large cucumber, quartered

½ pound Dungeness crabmeat

¼ cup Keto Mayonnaise (page 225)

1 to 2 tablespoons Low-Carb Ketchup (page 226)

1 or 2 dashes Tabasco, or other hot sauce

⅛ teaspoon smoked paprika

⅛ teaspoon chili powder

Salt

Freshly ground black pepper

Lemon wedges, for serving

1. Divide the lettuce, eggs, radishes, avocado, tomato, cucumber, and crab, and arrange on two plates.

2. In a small bowl, stir together the mayonnaise, ketchup, Tabasco, paprika, and chili powder. Season with salt and pepper. Spoon the dressing onto the salads or serve on the side. Serve with lemon wedges.

VARIATION 1 **SHRIMP LOUIE SALAD:** Use cooked shrimp instead of crabmeat.

VARIATION 2 **CRAB LOUIE WITH ASPARAGUS:** Many times, crab Louie salad is served with asparagus; for this salad, just add 4 or 5 steamed asparagus spears, chopped into bite-size pieces, to each serving.

PER SERVING: Calories: 504; Total carbs: 23g; **Net carbs: 14g, 17%;** **Total fat: 31g, 54%; Protein: 36g, 29%;** Fiber: 9g; Sugar: 8g

VARIATION 1: Calories: 491; Total carbs: 22g; **Net carbs: 13g, 16%;** **Total fat: 31g, 55%; Protein: 34g, 29%;** Fiber: 9g; Sugar: 8g

VARIATION 2: Calories: 508; Total carbs: 24g; **Net carbs: 14g, 17%;** **Total** fat: 31g, 54%; Protein: 36g, 29%; Fiber: 10g; Sugar: 8g

CRAB-STUFFED MUSHROOMS

These delectable little keto mushrooms are perfect for a party, and they're always a hit. **MAKES 6 SERVINGS**

PREP TIME: 15 minutes
COOK TIME: 20 minutes

1 pound crabmeat

1 egg, whisked

¼ cup cream cheese, at room temperature

3 tablespoons Keto Mayonnaise (page 225)

2 tablespoons finely chopped fresh chives

½ cup shredded Monterey Jack cheese

1 teaspoon garlic powder

Salt

Freshly ground black pepper

18 baby bella mushrooms, or white button mushrooms, stemmed (keep for another use)

PER SERVING (3 stuffed mushrooms):
Calories: 207; Total carbs: 5g;
Net carbs: 4g, 9%; Total fat: 11g, 45%;
Protein: 23g, 48%; Fiber: 1g; Sugar: 2g

VARIATION 1: Calories: 268;
Total carbs: 9g; **Net carbs: 5g, 12%;**
Total fat: 16g, 51%; Protein: 24g, 37%;
Fiber: 4g; Sugar: 3g

VARIATION 2: Calories: 248;
Total carbs: 5g; **Net carbs: 4g, 7%;**
Total fat: 16g, 56%; Protein: 23g, 37%;
Fiber: 1g; Sugar: 2g

1. Preheat the oven to 350°F.

2. In a large bowl, stir together the crabmeat, egg, cream cheese, mayonnaise, chives, Monterey Jack cheese, and garlic powder. Season with salt and pepper and mix well to combine.

3. Stuff each mushroom with about 1½ tablespoons of crab mixture and transfer to a baking sheet. Bake for 20 to 25 minutes or until the crab is slightly browned and the mushrooms are fork-tender. Refrigerate leftovers in an airtight container for up to 5 days. Reheat in a 350°F oven for about 15 minutes or until warm.

VARIATION 1 **AVOCADO CRAB-STUFFED MUSHROOMS:** Add 1 ripe avocado to the crab mixture. Stir well to combine until smooth. Follow the rest of the recipe as written.

VARIATION 2 **CHICKEN-STUFFED MUSHROOMS:** If you're not in the mood for seafood use canned chicken instead of crab.

PERFECT PAIR: These are great as a starter with Grilled Soy Lime Flank Steak (page 105).

CLAM CHOWDER

If it's clam chowder you crave, it's easy to make it keto—just skip the potatoes you usually find in the recipe. This homemade version comes together pretty fast, and it's really delicious. The recipe calls for canned clams, so if you have them in your pantry chances are you're ready to go! Just a few vegetables, some butter, and lots of cream bring this hearty soup to life. **MAKES 5 SERVINGS**

PREP TIME: 10 minutes
COOK TIME: 25 minutes

6 tablespoons butter, divided

1 white onion, diced

1 garlic clove, minced

3 or 4 carrots, peeled and diced

2 celery stalks, diced

Salt

Freshly ground black pepper

4 cups chicken broth

2 bay leaves

3 (6.5-ounce) cans minced clams

1 cup heavy (whipping) cream

2 to 3 tablespoons chopped fresh parsley leaves

PER SERVING: Calories: 503;
Total carbs: 16g; **Net carbs: 14g, 12%;**
Total fat: 35g, 60%; Protein: 34g, 28%;
Fiber: 2g; Sugar: 3g

VARIATION 1: Calories: 428;
Total carbs: 10g; **Net carbs: 8g, 9%;**
Total fat: 34g, 69%; Protein: 23g, 22%;
Fiber: 2g; Sugar: 3g

VARIATION 2: Calories: 350;
Total carbs: 15g; **Net carbs: 13g, 15%;**
Total fat: 17g, 44%; Protein: 34g, 41%;
Fiber: 2g; Sugar: 3g

1. In a large saucepan over medium heat, melt 2 tablespoons of butter.

2. Add the onion and garlic. Sauté for 5 to 7 minutes until the onion is softened and translucent.

3. Add the remaining 4 tablespoons of butter along with the carrots and celery. Cook for 5 to 7 minutes more until the carrots and celery soften. Season with salt and pepper.

4. Stir in the chicken broth and bring the liquid to a simmer. Add the bay leaves.

5. Add the clams with their juices and stir to combine. Reduce the heat to low and pour in the cream. Season with salt and pepper. Simmer for 10 minutes more and ladle the soup into bowls, topping with the fresh parsley.

VARIATION 1 **SEAFOOD CHOWDER:** Instead of just clams, add ½ pound shrimp and ½ pound diced whitefish to the soup.

VARIATION 2 **NONDAIRY CLAM CHOWDER:** Skip the cream and use 5 cups chicken broth to make this soup nondairy.

COCONUT SHRIMP

I had never eaten coconut shrimp until I met my husband—he loves them and always ordered them at a restaurant we would occasionally go to in our college days. When I first went Paleo, my mom and I tried to make a Paleo version that ended up being really good on our first try. With just a few ingredients and about 30 minutes you, too, can have these delicious, succulent coconut shrimp on your table. **MAKES 4 SERVINGS**

PREP TIME: 15 minutes
COOK TIME: 15 minutes

1½ pounds shrimp, peeled (keep the tails on) and deveined

2 eggs

1 tablespoon tapioca starch, or arrowroot powder (optional)

1 cup shredded unsweetened coconut

Salt

Freshly ground black pepper

1 tablespoon coconut oil

PER SERVING: Calories: 342; Total carbs: 5g; **Net carbs: 3g, 6%;** **Total fat: 18g, 46%; Protein: 39g, 48%;** Fiber: 2g; Sugar: 1g

VARIATION 1: Calories: 345; Total carbs: 5g; **Net carbs: 3g, 6%;** **Total fat: 18g, 46%; Protein: 39g, 48%;** Fiber: 2g; Sugar: 1g

VARIATION 2: Calories: 342; Total carbs: 5g; **Net carbs: 3g, 6%;** **Total fat: 18g, 46%; Protein: 39g, 48%;** Fiber: 2g; Sugar: 1g

1. Butterfly the shrimp by slicing them down the back so they open a bit.

2. In a shallow bowl, whisk the eggs and tapioca starch (if using).

3. Pour the coconut into a second shallow bowl.

4. Dip the shrimp first into the egg mixture and then into the coconut, making sure the shrimp are well coated. Season with salt and pepper.

5. In a large skillet over medium-high heat, heat the coconut oil.

6. Add the coated shrimp and fry for 2 to 3 minutes per side or until the shrimp are pink and the coconut is lightly browned. Refrigerate leftovers in an airtight container for up to 3 days. Reheat in a skillet over medium heat.

VARIATION 1 **SPICY COCONUT SHRIMP:** Add 1 to 2 teaspoons ground cayenne pepper to the coconut.

VARIATION 2 **OVEN-BAKED COCONUT SHRIMP:** Instead of panfrying, arrange the coated shrimp on a baking sheet and bake at 400°F for 5 to 7 minutes or until the coconut is golden brown and the shrimp are pink and opaque.

GAMBAS AL AJILLO

When my husband and I lived in Charlotte, North Carolina, nearly every Friday we would go to this place called Zen Fusion for happy hour—they had awesome Asian- and Spanish-inspired tapas, and we'd get dumplings, sushi, and these gambas al ajillo, which came out in a little cast-iron skillet full of hot oil and sizzling shrimp and garlic. Now that we're on the other side of the country I make them at home, but they're just as delicious. **MAKES 4 SERVINGS (OR MORE AS AN APPETIZER)**

PREP TIME: 10 minutes
COOK TIME: 10 minutes

½ cup extra-virgin olive oil

10 to 12 garlic cloves, thinly sliced

1 pound jumbo shrimp,
tails removed

Salt

Freshly ground black pepper

PER SERVING: Calories: 370;
Total carbs: 4g; **Net carbs: 4g, 4%;**
Total fat: 29g, 69%; Protein: 24g, 27%;
Fiber: 0g; Sugar: 0g

VARIATION 1: Calories: 371;
Total carbs: 4g; **Net carbs: 4g, 4%;**
Total fat: 29g, 69%; Protein: 24g, 27%;
Fiber: 0g; Sugar: 0g

VARIATION 2: Calories: 350;
Total carbs: 5g; **Net carbs: 5g, 5%;**
Total fat: 28g, 71%; Protein: 20g, 24%;
Fiber: 0g; Sugar: 0g

1. In a large skillet over medium heat, heat the olive oil.

2. Add the garlic. Cook for 2 to 3 minutes until fragrant.

3. Add the shrimp and cook for 2 to 3 minutes per side until pink. Season with salt and pepper and serve right away. Refrigerate leftovers in an airtight container for up to 3 days.

VARIATION 1 **SPICY GAMBAS AL AJILLO:** Add 1 teaspoon red pepper flakes or ground cayenne pepper to the skillet before serving. Give everything a toss to combine well.

VARIATION 2 **SCALLOPS AL AJILLO:** Use scallops instead of shrimp. Cook in the olive oil over medium heat for 5 to 6 minutes per side.

PAN-SEARED SCALLOPS WITH LEMON BUTTER

Served with a big salad, this makes a fantastic dinner, or you could serve it as an appetizer or snack at a dinner party. Scallops and butter are so good together, and they're even better with a little lemon thrown in. **MAKES 4 SERVINGS**

PREP TIME: 10 minutes
COOK TIME: 20 minutes

1 pound scallops, rinsed under cold water and patted dry with a paper towel

Salt

Freshly ground black pepper

4 tablespoons butter, divided

1 lemon, halved

Zest of ½ lemon

PER SERVING: Calories: 200; Total carbs: 3g; **Net carbs: 3g, 5%;** **Total fat: 12g, 54%; Protein: 19g, 41%;** Fiber: 0g; Sugar: 0g

VARIATION 1: Calories: 201; Total carbs: 1g; **Net carbs: 1g, 2%;** **Total fat: 13g, 53%; Protein: 23g, 45%;** Fiber: 0g; Sugar: 0g

VARIATION 2: Calories: 201; Total carbs: 3g; **Net carbs: 3g, 5%;** **Total fat: 12g, 54%; Protein: 19g, 41%;** Fiber: 0g; Sugar: 0g

1. Season the scallops on both sides with salt and pepper.

2. In a large nonstick skillet over medium-high heat, melt 2 tablespoons of butter.

3. Add the scallops. Cook for 5 to 7 minutes per side or until the scallops begin to get crispy.

4. Squeeze 1 lemon half over the scallops. Transfer the scallops to a serving platter.

5. Return the skillet to low heat. Add the remaining 2 tablespoons of butter.

6. Stir in the lemon zest and squeeze the remaining lemon half into the skillet. Stir continuously until the butter reduces slightly, 4 to 5 minutes. Pour the sauce over the scallops and serve immediately. Refrigerate leftovers in an airtight container for up to 2 days.

VARIATION 1 **PAN-SEARED SHRIMP WITH LEMON BUTTER:** Use shrimp instead of scallops: Cook the shrimp for 2 to 3 minutes per side over medium-high heat.

VARIATION 2 **PAN-SEARED SCALLOPS WITH ROSEMARY LEMON BUTTER:** Add 1 tablespoon chopped fresh rosemary leaves to the butter sauce before serving.

ALLERGEN TIP: If you're allergic to shellfish, pan-sear diced whitefish, such as cod, for 2 to 3 minutes per side, and serve with the lemon butter sauce.

LOW-CARB LOWCOUNTRY SEAFOOD BOIL

One of my favorite dinners to make in summer is a seafood boil, especially when we have a lot of people over. It does take some time, but it's always a huge hit and a really fun way to feed a crowd. My brother and I have a recipe we've perfected over the years. Usually it includes potatoes and corn, but I omit them here to keep it keto-friendly. **MAKES 8 SERVINGS**

PREP TIME: 1 hour
COOK TIME: 1 hour

4 gallons water

6 bay leaves

2 onions, quartered

2 lemons, halved

3 tablespoons salt

2½ tablespoons paprika

1½ tablespoons ground coriander

1 tablespoon ground allspice

1 tablespoon red pepper flakes

1 tablespoon chili powder

1 tablespoon dried marjoram

1 tablespoon onion powder

1 tablespoon garlic powder

1 tablespoon dry mustard

1 tablespoon dried tarragon

1 tablespoon dried thyme

1 tablespoon dried rosemary

2½ teaspoons peppercorns

1 teaspoon ground cumin

½ teaspoon ground cayenne pepper

2 pounds Italian sausage, each link cut into thirds

1½ pounds mussels

2½ pounds cod fillets

3½ pounds snow crab legs

1½ pounds large raw shrimp, shells on

1. Fill a large stockpot over high heat about three-fourths full with the water. Bring to a boil. Add the bay leaves, onions, lemons, salt, paprika, coriander, allspice, red pepper flakes, chili powder, marjoram, onion powder, garlic powder, mustard, tarragon, thyme, rosemary, peppercorns, cumin, and cayenne.

2. In a large skillet over medium heat, cook the sausage for about 3 minutes per side, turning to brown all sides. They don't have to be fully cooked because they'll finish cooking in the stockpot. Remove from the heat and set aside.

3. Remove any excess fat from the skillet and place it back over medium heat. Add the mussels and 1 cup of seasoned water from the stockpot. Cover the skillet and steam the mussels for 5 to 7 minutes. Discard any that don't open.

4. Add the sausage to the stockpot, followed by the cod. Keep the water at a low boil and cook for 5 minutes.

5. Add the mussels and crab legs. Cook for 5 minutes more.

6. About 5 minutes before you're ready to serve, add the shrimp. Cook for 4 to 5 minutes until completely pink and opaque.

7. Carefully drain the contents of the stockpot and transfer everything to a large serving bowl. Serve immediately. Go traditional and pour the contents of the bowl onto a newspaper-lined table and dig in with your hands! ➤

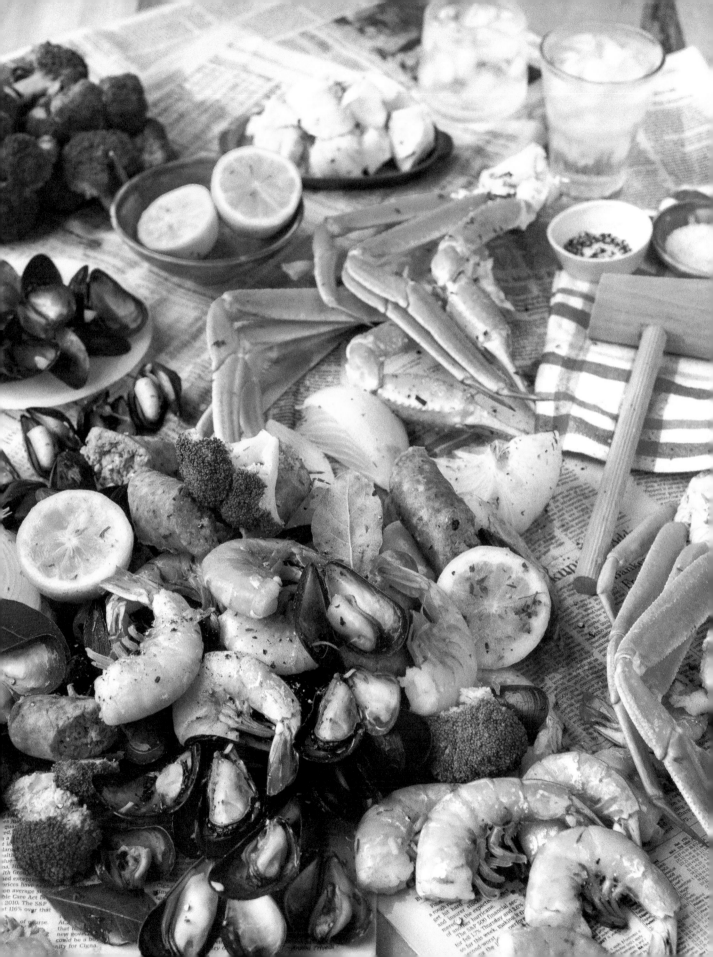

PER SERVING: Calories: 805; Total carbs: 7g; **Net carbs: 7g, 4%; Total fat: 40g, 45%; Protein: 96g, 51%;** Fiber: 0g; Sugar: 1g

VARIATION 1: Calories: 795; Total carbs: 6g; **Net carbs: 6g, 3%; Total fat: 39g, 45%; Protein: 97g, 52%;** Fiber: 0g; Sugar: 1g

VARIATION 2: Calories: 814; Total carbs: 9g; **Net carbs: 8g, 4%; Total fat: 41g, 45%; Protein: 97g, 51%;** Fiber: 1g; Sugar: 2g

VARIATION 1 **SEAFOOD BOIL WITH CLAMS:** For a variation on some of the shellfish, use clams instead of mussels. I actually prefer clams to mussels, but they are usually more expensive so I don't use them as often. (This recipe is great because you can use whatever seafood you like—feel free to add or omit as you please.)

VARIATION 2 **SEAFOOD BOIL WITH VEGGIES:** Get some extra veggies in by adding a head of chopped broccoli or cauliflower to the stockpot when you add the mussels and crab.

CREAMY SHRIMP AND BACON SKILLET

Shrimp and bacon are two things you might not immediately think of combining (unless you've made my Bacon-Wrapped Shrimp, see Variation 2 on page 28), but the two are so delicious when paired that I find myself coming up with dishes that incorporate both as often as possible. This one-pot meal is great on its own or with some zucchini noodles, served with a side salad. It could also be served in a smaller portion as the first course of a larger meal. **MAKES 4 SERVINGS**

PREP TIME: 5 minutes
COOK TIME: 20 minutes

10 ounces thick-cut bacon, diced

½ onion, diced

2 garlic cloves, minced

1 pound shrimp, peeled, deveined, tails removed

Salt

Freshly ground black pepper

4 ounces cream cheese

Dash chicken broth (optional)

¼ cup grated Parmesan cheese

PER SERVING: Calories: 574; Total carbs: 5g; **Net carbs: 5g, 4%;** **Total fat: 45g, 70%; Protein: 36g, 26%;** Fiber: 0g; Sugar: 2g

VARIATION 1: Calories: 587; Total carbs: 7g; **Net carbs: 6g, 4%;** **Total fat: 45g, 69%; Protein: 27g, 27%;** Fiber: 1g; Sugar: 2g

VARIATION 2: Calories: 578; Total carbs: 5g; **Net carbs: 4g, 3%;** **Total fat: 45g, 70%; Protein: 36g, 27%;** Fiber: 1g; Sugar: 2g

1. Preheat the broiler.

2. In a large ovenproof skillet over medium-high heat, cook the bacon in its own fat for about 5 minutes until it starts to get crispy.

3. Add the onion and garlic. Sauté for 5 to 7 minutes until the onion is softened and translucent.

4. Add the shrimp. Season with salt and pepper. Cook for 2 to 3 minutes, stirring, or until the shrimp start to turn pink.

5. Add the cream cheese and stir well to combine as it melts. If necessary, add a splash of chicken broth to thin it out.

6. Top with the Parmesan and transfer the skillet to the oven. Broil for 4 to 5 minutes until the Parmesan is lightly browned. Refrigerate leftovers in an airtight container for up to 5 days.

VARIATION 1 **CREAMY SHRIMP AND BACON SKILLET WITH MUSHROOMS:** Add about 8 ounces sliced mushrooms to the skillet after the onion and garlic. Cook for 5 to 6 minutes or until they start to brown. Add the shrimp and follow the rest of the recipe as written.

VARIATION 2 **CREAMY SHRIMP AND BACON SKILLET WITH SPINACH:** Add 2 cups chopped fresh spinach to the skillet after the shrimp is cooked. Stir well to combine as it wilts. Follow the rest of the recipe as written.

PERFECT PAIR: Serve this dish over Old-School Buttered (Zucchini) Noodles (page 218) to make it a low-carb pasta dinner!

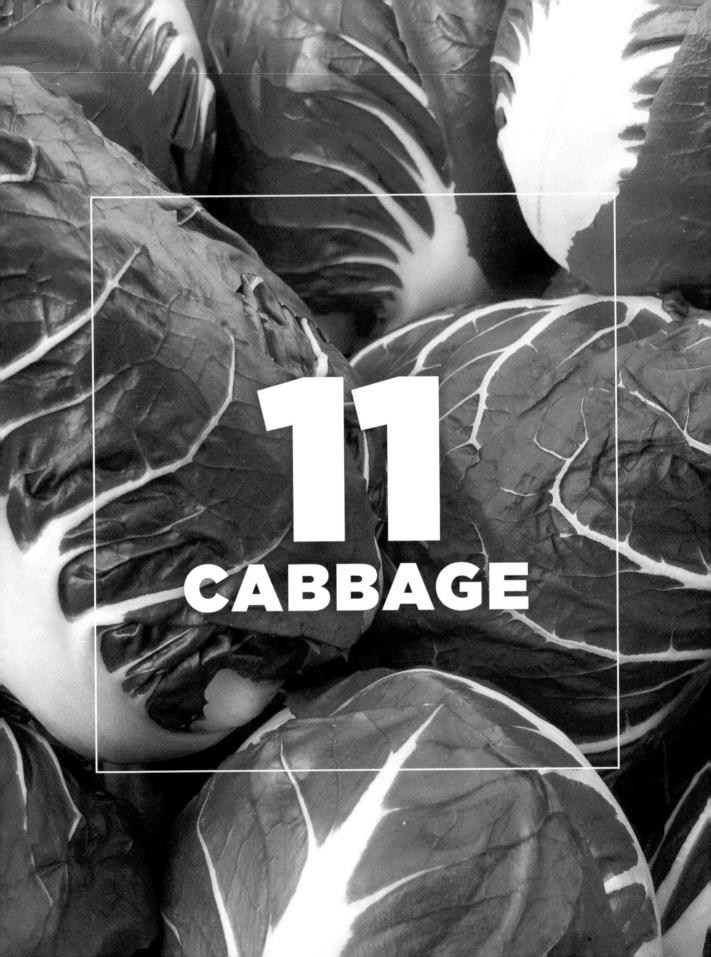

11
CABBAGE

Cabbage is a great keto vegetable because it's very low in carbs and incredibly versatile in texture and flavor—you can steam it, fry it, sauté it, roast it—and it does well as a wrap substitute (Keto Asian Dumplings, page 152, and Roast Beef Cabbage Wraps, page 154). There are several kinds of cabbage, and most of them last a long time in the refrigerator, which I appreciate—I always end up buying too much lettuce and it goes a bit wilty before I can use it all, but that never seems to be the case with cabbage.

This chapter is one of my favorites because it spans cheesy comfort food to grain-free Asian dumplings. I've even included my favorite quick lunch recipe (Roast Beef Cabbage Wraps, page 154).

KETO ASIAN DUMPLINGS

I love Chinese food more than pretty much anything, and out of all the delicious dishes to choose from, dumplings of any kind are probably my favorite. Unfortunately there's nothing low-carb about them, so I made these keto Asian dumplings—succulent dumpling filling wrapped in steamed cabbage and dipped in a spicy sesame vinaigrette. **MAKES 4 SERVINGS**

PREP TIME: 20 minutes
COOK TIME: 20 minutes

FOR THE DIPPING SAUCE
¼ cup gluten-free soy sauce
2 tablespoons sesame oil
1 tablespoon rice vinegar
1 teaspoon chili garlic sauce

FOR THE FILLING
1 tablespoon sesame oil
2 garlic cloves
1 teaspoon grated fresh ginger
1 celery stalk, minced
½ onion, minced
1 carrot, minced
8 ounces ground pork
8 ounces shrimp, peeled, deveined, and finely chopped
2 tablespoons gluten-free soy sauce
½ teaspoon fish sauce
Salt
Freshly ground black pepper
3 scallions, green parts only, chopped
1 head napa cabbage, rinsed, leaves separated (about 12 leaves)

TO MAKE THE DIPPING SAUCE

1. In a small bowl, whisk together the soy sauce, sesame oil, vinegar, and chili garlic sauce. Set aside.

TO MAKE THE FILLING

1. In a large skillet over medium heat, heat the sesame oil.

2. Add the garlic, ginger, celery, onion, and carrot. Sauté for 5 to 7 minutes until softened.

3. Add the pork. Cook for 5 to 6 minutes, breaking it up with a spoon, until it starts to brown.

4. Add the shrimp and stir everything together well.

5. Stir in the soy sauce and fish sauce. Season with a little salt and pepper. Give it a stir and add the scallions. Keep it warm over low heat until ready to fill the dumplings.

6. Steam the cabbage leaves: Place the leaves in a large saucepan with just 1 to 2 inches of boiling water. Cook for about 5 minutes or until the leaves become tender. Remove from the water and set aside to drain.

7. Lay each leaf out flat. Put about 2 tablespoons of filling in the center of one leaf. Wrap the leaf over itself, tucking the sides in so the whole thing is tightly wrapped. Secure with a toothpick. Continue with the remaining leaves and filling. Serve with the dipping sauce. Refrigerate leftovers in an airtight container for up to 3 days.

VARIATION 1 **PORK DUMPLINGS:** Skip the shrimp and double the amount of pork.

VARIATION 2 **VEGETARIAN DUMPLINGS:** Use 1 pound mushrooms, diced, instead of pork and shrimp.

PERFECT PAIR: Serve these with a side of Asian Cauliflower Fried Rice (see page 178).

ROAST BEEF CABBAGE WRAPS

For as long as I've been Paleo, I've been wrapping lunch meat in lettuce and calling it a day, but a few months ago I realized that cabbage leaves were not only sturdier, but also lasted longer in my refrigerator (I'm notorious for forgetting about lettuce and having to throw half of it away). So now I almost exclusively use cabbage for low-carb wraps—I can stuff more into them, which means I only have to make one or two instead of my usual three to four lettuce wraps. **MAKES 4 SERVINGS**

PREP TIME: 5 minutes
COOK TIME: 0 minutes

   30 DF GF NF

12 ounces sliced roast beef

2 to 3 tablespoons yellow mustard

2 to 3 tablespoons Keto Mayonnaise (page 225)

4 thin slices tomato

4 thin slices red onion

4 large cabbage leaves, washed, dried, tough end stemmed

PER SERVING: Calories: 200; Total carbs: 5g; **Net carbs: 4g, 8%;** **Total fat: 10g, 44%; Protein: 23g, 48%;** Fiber: 1g; Sugar: 3g

VARIATION 1: Calories: 313; Total carbs: 5g; **Net carbs: 4g, 6%;** **Total fat: 19g, 54%; Protein: 30g, 40%;** Fiber: 1g; Sugar: 3g

VARIATION 2: Calories: 224; Total carbs: 10g; **Net carbs: 4g, 16%;** **Total fat: 9g, 32%; Protein: 28g, 54%;** Fiber: 6g; Sugar: 4g

Assemble each wrap: Layer roast beef, mustard, mayonnaise, tomato, and red onion on each leaf and wrap it up like a tortilla, tucking the thinner end of the leaf in so the fillings don't fall out. Serve immediately.

VARIATION 1 **ROAST BEEF CABBAGE WRAPS WITH CHEESE:** Add 1 slice pepper jack or Cheddar to each wrap.

VARIATION 2 **TURKEY CLUB CABBAGE WRAPS:** Instead of roast beef and red onion, use turkey, sliced avocado, and some lettuce for each wrap.

ASIAN SLAW

This is a great recipe for days when maybe you feel like having Chinese food but don't want to spend much time cooking, and definitely don't want to stray from keto enough to order takeout! I love the combination of napa cabbage with sesame oil, tangy vinegar, and crunchy almonds—and this recipe actually incorporates some veggies as well, so you get a little red bell pepper and sliced carrot. I love it on its own or with some grilled chicken thrown in. **MAKES 4 SERVINGS**

PREP TIME: 15 minutes
COOK TIME: 0 minutes

1 head napa cabbage, thinly sliced

½ red bell pepper, julienned

½ carrot, julienned

¼ cup sliced almonds

¼ cup sesame oil

3 tablespoons rice wine vinegar

Juice of 1 lime

Salt

Freshly ground black pepper

1 teaspoon red pepper flakes

2 scallions, green parts only, sliced

2 tablespoons sesame seeds

Chopped fresh cilantro, for garnish

1. In a large bowl, combine the cabbage, bell pepper, carrot, and almonds.

2. In a small bowl, whisk together the sesame oil, vinegar, and lime juice. Season with salt and pepper. Stir in the red pepper flakes. Pour the dressing over the veggie mixture and toss well to combine.

3. Sprinkle with the scallions and sesame seeds. Toss again. Garnish with cilantro before serving.

VARIATION 1 **ASIAN SLAW WITH PEANUT DRESSING:** Add 2 tablespoons unsweetened peanut butter to the dressing. Add 3 tablespoons crushed peanuts as a garnish along with the cilantro.

VARIATION 2 **ASIAN SLAW WITH AVOCADO:** Add 1 avocado, diced, to the slaw for some extra fat.

PERFECT PAIR: Serve this slaw as a side with Classic Roast Pork Tenderloin (page 117).

PER SERVING: Calories: 229;
Total carbs: 8g; **Net carbs: 4g, 14%;**
Total fat: 21g, 80%; Protein: 5g, 6%;
Fiber: 4g; Sugar: 3g

VARIATION 1: Calories: 361;
Total carbs: 12g; **Net carbs: 7g, 13%;**
Total fat: 32g, 77%; Protein: 11g, 10%;
Fiber: 5g; Sugar: 4g

VARIATION 2: Calories: 320;
Total carbs: 14g; **Net carbs: 6g, 17%;**
Total fat: 29g, 77%; Protein: 6g, 6%;
Fiber: 8g; Sugar: 5g

STUFFED CABBAGE ROLLS

These stuffed cabbage rolls feel so old school to me, as comforting as a casserole or lasagna, but they're low-carb and grain-free and a perfect keto dinner. The combination of ground beef and sausage with onion and just enough tomato sauce is so satisfying. **MAKES 8 SERVINGS**

PREP TIME: 20 minutes
COOK TIME: 1 hour, 30 minutes

1 large head cabbage, separated into 16 leaves

1 pound ground beef

1 pound sausage

1 small onion, chopped

2 garlic cloves, minced

Salt

Freshly ground black pepper

1 cup chicken broth

½ cup canned no-sugar-added tomato sauce, warmed

Grated Parmesan cheese, for topping

PER SERVING (2 rolls): Calories: 331; Total carbs: 11g; **Net carbs: 7g, 12%; Total fat: 23g, 61%; Protein: 22g, 27%;** Fiber: 4g; Sugar: 6g

VARIATION 1: Calories: 331; Total carbs: 11g; **Net carbs: 7g, 12%; Total fat: 23g, 61%; Protein: 22g, 27%;** Fiber: 4g; Sugar: 6g

VARIATION 2: Calories: 388; Total carbs:11 g; **Net carbs: 7g, 10%; Total fat:27 g, 63%; Protein: 26g, 27%;** Fiber: 4g; Sugar: 6g

1. Bring a large saucepan of water to a boil over high heat. Add the cabbage leaves and boil for 2 to 3 minutes or until soft. Remove from the water and set aside to drain. Discard the water.

2. In a large bowl, mix together the beef, sausage, onion, and garlic. Season well with salt and pepper. Spoon the meat mixture into each leaf and fold the sides over, rolling each leaf up to hold the meat mixture. Secure with a toothpick and transfer to the pan.

3. Add the chicken broth. Cover the pan and simmer over low heat for about 1 hour, 30 minutes or until the meat is cooked through. Remove the rolls from the broth and top with the warmed tomato sauce and a sprinkle of Parmesan. Refrigerate leftovers in an airtight container for up to 3 days.

VARIATION 1 **BAKED STUFFED CABBAGE ROLLS:** Follow the recipe as written but transfer the rolls to a large baking dish with a lid. Add the chicken broth, cover the dish, and bake at 350°F for about 1 hour. Top with the tomato sauce and Parmesan before serving.

VARIATION 2 **CHEESY STUFFED CABBAGE ROLLS:** Add 1 cup shredded Cheddar to the meat mixture.

CABBAGE CASSEROLE

This casserole is a great way to get more veggies into your diet—the cabbage blends right in and goes so well with the meat and sauces. If this weren't a keto recipe I would add a cup of white rice, but it's just as satisfying without any added carbs. **MAKES 4 SERVINGS**

PREP TIME: 10 minutes
COOK TIME: 35 minutes

 GF NF

1 tablespoon olive oil

¼ white onion, diced

½ pound ground beef

½ pound ground pork

Salt

Freshly ground black pepper

2 eggs

½ cup heavy (whipping) cream

2 tablespoons tomato paste

1 cup shredded provolone cheese, divided

1 large head cabbage, shredded

PER SERVING: Calories: 650; Total carbs: 22g; **Net carbs: 14g, 12%;** **Total fat: 48g, 66%; Protein: 36g, 22%;** Fiber: 8g; Sugar: 11g

VARIATION 1: Calories: 714; Total carbs: 22g; **Net carbs: 14g, 11%;** **Total fat: 56g, 70%; Protein: 34g, 19%;** Fiber: 8g; Sugar: 11g

VARIATION 2: Calories: 651; Total carbs: 22g; **Net carbs: 14g, 12%;** **Total fat: 48g, 66%; Protein: 36g, 22%;** Fiber: 8g; Sugar: 12g

1. Preheat the oven to 350°F.

2. In a large skillet over medium heat, heat the olive oil.

3. Add the onion. Sauté for 5 to 7 minutes until softened and translucent.

4. Add the beef and pork. Cook for 5 to 7 minutes until browned. Season with salt and pepper. Drain off the grease and transfer the meat mixture to a 7-by-11-inch baking dish.

5. In a medium bowl, whisk together the eggs, cream, tomato paste, and ½ cup of provolone. Season with salt and pepper.

6. Top the meat mixture with the shredded cabbage and pour the egg mixture over it. Gently shake the dish and tap it on the counter to ensure the mixture makes it through to the bottom and sides of the dish. Top with the remaining ½ cup of provolone. Bake for 25 minutes until the cheese melts and the corners are set and bubbling slightly. Cover and refrigerate leftovers for up to 3 days.

VARIATION 1 **SPICY ITALIAN SAUSAGE CABBAGE CASSEROLE:** Instead of ground beef and pork, use 1 pound hot Italian sausage, chopped. Swap out the provolone for mozzarella and follow the rest of the recipe as written.

VARIATION 2 **SPINACH AND CABBAGE CASSEROLE:** Add some extra greens by throwing 1 cup chopped fresh spinach into the casserole with the cabbage.

SPICY SAUSAGE AND CABBAGE SKILLET

Spicy sausage and cabbage is such a delicious combination, and this recipe is a winner because it's a one-pot dinner. My favorite recipes tend to be those cooked in cast-iron skillets that you sauté on the stove and then finish in the oven, giving you time to clean up the kitchen a bit before serving, so when it's time to eat you can just enjoy your food and your company. **MAKES 4 SERVINGS**

PREP TIME: 5 minutes
COOK TIME: 35 minutes

1 tablespoon olive oil

1 small white onion, diced

1 garlic clove, minced

1 pound hot Italian sausage, casings removed

1 head cabbage, chopped

Salt

Freshly ground black pepper

1 cup shredded provolone cheese

PER SERVING: Calories: 602; Total carbs: 17g; **Net carbs: 11g, 10%; Total fat: 48g, 71%; Protein: 28g, 19%;** Fiber: 6g; Sugar: 8g

VARIATION 1: Calories: 555; Total carbs: 16g; **Net carbs: 10g, 10%; Total fat: 43g, 69%; Protein: 29g, 21%;** Fiber: 6g; Sugar: 8g

VARIATION 2: Calories: 694; Total carbs: 23g; **Net carbs: 13g, 12%; Total fat: 56g, 71%; Protein: 29g, 17%;** Fiber: 10g; Sugar: 10g

1. Preheat the oven to 350°F.

2. In a large cast-iron skillet over medium heat, heat the olive oil.

3. Add the onion and garlic. Sauté for 5 to 7 minutes until the onion is softened and translucent.

4. Add the sausage and cook for 7 to 10 minutes or until browned. Remove from the heat, slice the sausage, and return it to the skillet.

5. Add the cabbage and season with salt and pepper.

6. Top with the provolone and transfer the skillet to the oven. Bake for 20 minutes or until the cheese melts. Refrigerate leftovers in an airtight container for up to 6 days.

VARIATION 1 **CHICKEN SAUSAGE AND CABBAGE SKILLET:** Use chicken sausage instead of hot Italian (or use mild Italian sausage).

VARIATION 2 **SAUSAGE AND CABBAGE SKILLET WITH AVOCADO:** Add 1 large avocado, diced, to the skillet before serving. Garnish with chopped scallions.

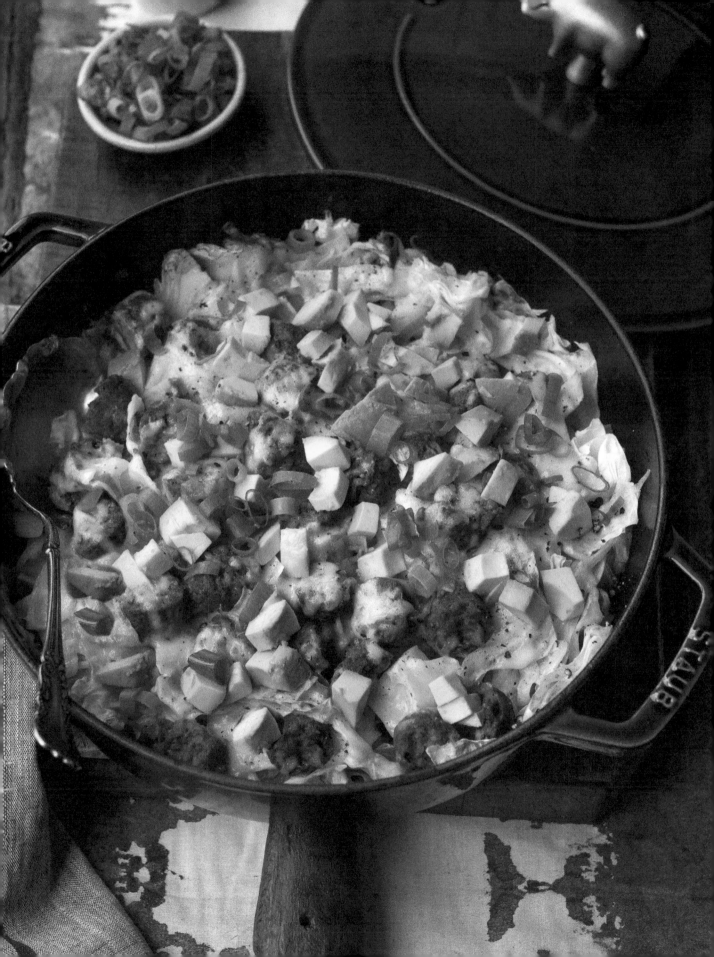

KETO COLESLAW

Coleslaw is a great snack or side that's pretty keto on it's own, and you don't have to do anything special to it to make it a low-carb dish. I love this one with ribs, as a side with chicken or steak, or even just on its own as a quick snack. You could easily add some other spices to add variety to the flavor, but I like this classic, straightforward recipe. **MAKES 4 SERVINGS**

PREP TIME: 15 minutes
COOK TIME: 0 minutes

10 ounces shredded cabbage

¼ red onion, diced

½ cup Keto Mayonnaise (page 225)

1 tablespoon red wine vinegar

1 teaspoon dry mustard

1 teaspoon celery seed

Salt

Freshly ground black pepper

PER SERVING: Calories: 140; Total carbs: 12g; **Net carbs: 10g, 33%; Total fat: 10g, 64%; Protein: 2g, 3%;** Fiber: 2g; Sugar: 2g

VARIATION 1: Calories: 149; Total carbs: 13g; **Net carbs: 11g, 36%; Total fat: 10g, 61%; Protein: 2g, 4%;** Fiber: 2g; Sugar: 2g

VARIATION 2: Calories: 140; Total carbs: 12g; **Net carbs: 10g, 33%; Total fat: 10g, 64%; Protein: 2g, 3%;** Fiber: 2g; Sugar: 2g

In a large bowl, combine the cabbage, red onion, mayonnaise, vinegar, mustard, and celery seed. Season with salt and pepper and mix well to combine. Serve immediately or cover and refrigerate for up to 1 week.

VARIATION 1 **KALE AND CABBAGE COLESLAW:** Add 1 cup stemmed and chopped kale leaves. You may need to add a few more tablespoons of mayonnaise and another splash of vinegar. Toss well to combine and serve.

VARIATION 2 **KETO COLESLAW WITH RED CABBAGE:** Add 1 cup shredded red cabbage to the mix. If necessary, add a few more tablespoons of mayonnaise and another splash of vinegar. Toss well to combine and serve.

CABBAGE SOUP

This cabbage soup is one of those "everything in the refrigerator" kind of meals, which I love because it's a fantastic way to use up any veggies that might be on their way out. Plus, it's delicious and packed with vegetables, which I sometimes don't get enough of every day. I like adding a cup of this soup as a side with lunch and dinner. **MAKES 6 SERVINGS**

PREP TIME: 20 minutes
COOK TIME: 30 minutes

1 tablespoon olive oil

3 garlic cloves, minced

1 onion, diced

3 carrots, diced

1 celery stalk, diced

½ green bell pepper, diced

Salt

Freshly ground black pepper

1 cup chopped kale

2 tablespoons tomato paste

2 (32-ounce) cartons chicken broth

1 large head cabbage, chopped

1 teaspoon dried oregano

1 teaspoon dried thyme

Grated Parmesan cheese, for topping

PER SERVING: Calories: 156; Total carbs: 23g; **Net carbs: 16g, 51%; Total fat: 5g, 26%; Protein: 10g, 23%;** Fiber: 7g; Sugar: 10g

VARIATION 1: Calories: 385; Total carbs: 23g; **Net carbs: 14g, 20%; Total fat: 25g, 58%; Protein: 22g, 22%;** Fiber: 7g; Sugar: 10g

VARIATION 2: Calories: 153; Total carbs: 23g; **Net carbs: 16g, 51%; Total fat: 5g, 27%; Protein: 9g, 22%;** Fiber: 7g; Sugar: 10g

1. In a large saucepan over medium heat, heat the olive oil.

2. Add the garlic and onion. Sauté for 5 minutes.

3. Add the carrots and celery. Cook for 5 to 7 minutes until softened.

4. Add the bell pepper and stir well to combine. Cook for 5 to 7 minutes more. Season with salt and pepper and add the kale.

5. Stir in the tomato paste until well combined.

6. Pour in the chicken broth and bring the soup to a gentle boil.

7. Add the cabbage, oregano, and thyme. Season with more salt and pepper. Reduce the heat to low, cover the pan, and simmer for 15 minutes (a little longer if you have the time). Ladle into bowls and top with Parmesan before serving.

VARIATION 1 **SAUSAGE AND CABBAGE SOUP:** Add 1 pound spicy sausage to the saucepan with the veggies. Cook for another 5 minutes or until browned. Follow the rest of the recipe as written.

VARIATION 2 **VEGETARIAN CABBAGE SOUP:** Use vegetable broth instead of chicken broth to make this soup vegetarian.

MAKE IT PALEO: Skip the Parmesan to keep this Paleo and dairy-free.

CREAMED CABBAGE

This is an easy side dish you can throw together in no time, as long as you've got the cabbage in your refrigerator; you probably have all the other ingredients as well! I like it as a side with steak or chicken, or even as a tasty snack on its own. **MAKES 4 SERVINGS**

PREP TIME: 10 minutes
COOK TIME: 20 minutes

2 tablespoons butter

1 garlic clove, minced

1 cup heavy (whipping) cream

Salt

Freshly ground black pepper

¼ cup grated Parmesan cheese

1 large head cabbage, shredded

¼ cup shredded provolone cheese

PER SERVING: Calories: 390;
Total carbs: 20g; **Net carbs: 12g, 19%;**
Total fat: 32g, 72%; Protein: 10g, 9%;
Fiber: 8g; Sugar: 10g

VARIATION 1: Calories: 390;
Total carbs: 20g; **Net carbs: 12g, 19%;**
Total fat: 32g, 72%; Protein: 10g, 9%;
Fiber: 8g; Sugar: 10g

VARIATION 2: Calories: 597;
Total carbs: 21g; **Net carbs: 13g, 13%;**
Total fat: 52g, 77%; Protein: 16g, 10%;
Fiber: 8g; Sugar: 10g

1. In a large saucepan over medium heat, melt the butter.

2. Add the garlic and sauté for 2 to 3 minutes until fragrant.

3. Add the cream and bring to a simmer. Season with salt and pepper.

4. While stirring, slowly add the Parmesan.

5. Add the cabbage and cook for 5 to 7 minutes or until tender. Season with more salt and pepper.

6. Top with the provolone and let it melt, stirring occasionally. Serve warm. Refrigerate leftovers in an airtight container for up to 4 days.

VARIATION 1 **OVEN-BAKED CREAMED CABBAGE:** Bring about 1 inch of water to a boil in a large saucepan. Add the cabbage and cook for 2 to 3 minutes until softened. In an 8- or 9-inch square baking dish, combine the garlic, melted butter, cream, and Parmesan. Add the cabbage and stir well. Top with the provolone and bake at 350°F for about 20 minutes.

VARIATION 2 **CREAMED CABBAGE WITH PANCETTA:** Instead of butter, panfry 8 ounces diced pancetta in the saucepan over medium-high heat for 5 to 7 minutes. Add the garlic and follow the rest of the recipe as written.

SOUTHERN FRIED CABBAGE

This southern fried cabbage is an awesome side dish recipe to have in your back pocket. With just a few ingredients, it provides lots of flavor and is always a hit at a potluck party or barbecue, or even just as a side dish for your next Sunday dinner. Recipes that start with bacon and use its fat to cook the rest of the ingredients result in such flavorful dishes. **MAKES 4 SERVINGS**

PREP TIME: 10 minutes
COOK TIME: 15 minutes

3 bacon slices, diced

1 small white onion, diced

1 garlic clove, minced

1 head cabbage, chopped

Salt

Freshly ground black pepper

PER SERVING: Calories: 161; Total carbs: 15g; **Net carbs: 9g, 35%;** **Total fat: 10g, 54%; Protein: 6g, 11%;** Fiber: 6g; Sugar: 8g

VARIATION 1: Calories: 352; Total carbs: 16g; **Net carbs: 10g, 17%;** **Total fat: 28g, 71%; Protein: 12g, 12%;** Fiber: 6g; Sugar: 8g

VARIATION 2: Calories: 154; Total carbs: 15g; **Net carbs: 9g, 36%;** **Total fat: 10g, 59%; Protein: 3g, 5%;** Fiber: 6g; Sugar: 8g

1. In a large saucepan over medium-high heat, sauté the bacon for 5 to 7 minutes until it begins to crisp.

2. Add the onion and garlic and sauté for 5 to 7 minutes until the onion is softened and translucent.

3. Add the cabbage, tossing it in the bacon fat. Season with salt and pepper and cook for about 5 minutes or until the cabbage softens and begins to brown and get a little crispy around the edges. Refrigerate leftovers in an airtight container for up to 3 days.

VARIATION 1 **SOUTHERN FRIED CABBAGE WITH EGG:** Make this a breakfast dish by serving with 1 or 2 fried eggs on top. In a skillet over medium-high heat, cook the eggs in 1 tablespoon butter or olive oil for 3 to 4 minutes. Gently flip and cook until the yolk is cooked to your preference.

VARIATION 2 **VEGETARIAN FRIED CABBAGE:** Use butter or olive oil instead of bacon to make this dish vegetarian.

PERFECT PAIR: Serve as a side with Uncle Marty's Chicken (page 90).

12
CAULIFLOWER

Cauliflower is a terrific substitute for so many carby things (rice, potatoes, even bread) because it has a starchy quality and adapts to a wide variety of flavors easily. I'm sure by now you've seen more than enough recipes for cauliflower rice, but the truth is that you can do a lot more with cauliflower than just sauté it. For example, it makes an amazing low-carb pizza crust, really delicious mashed "fauxtatoes" (as I like to call them), and let's not forget how great it is without first running it through a food processor!

In this chapter you'll find a cheesy cauliflower gratin, some delicious roasted cauliflower, and a lot of keto substitutes for the usual grain- and carb-laden foods such as grilled cheese sandwiches, pizza, and even "tater" tots. Keep a head of cauliflower (or a bag of chopped florets) in your refrigerator all the time because you never know when a carb craving may strike, and cauliflower is the number-one ingredient to keep you on track when it happens.

CAULIFLOWER PIZZA

My husband and I first made this pizza on New Year's Day, 2017—we aren't usually big New Year's resolution people, but at that time, going keto was really important to us so we decided to do it together starting January 1. We watched *Breaking Bad* all day and took a lunch break to make this pizza before heading to Half Moon Bay to visit my side of the family—it's one of those food memories I probably won't ever forget. **MAKES 1 PIZZA**

PREP TIME: 15 minutes
COOK TIME: 35 minutes

Butter, or olive oil, for the baking dish

1 head cauliflower, chopped roughly into florets

½ cup shredded mozzarella cheese, plus more for topping

½ cup grated Parmesan cheese

1 teaspoon dried oregano

1 teaspoon dried thyme

1 teaspoon garlic powder

1 teaspoon onion powder

½ teaspoon red pepper flakes

1 tablespoon salt

Freshly ground black pepper

2 eggs, whisked

¼ cup sugar-free pizza sauce

10 ounces sliced pepperoni

1. Preheat the oven to 400°F.

2. Grease a baking sheet with butter. Set aside. Alternatively, use a pizza stone.

3. In a food processor, pulse the cauliflower until fine. Transfer to a microwave-safe container and microwave, uncovered, on high power for 2 minutes. Cool slightly. Place the cauliflower in a thin cloth or piece of cheesecloth and twist to remove any water (not a lot will come out but the little that's there needs to be removed). Transfer to a large bowl.

4. Add the mozzarella, Parmesan, oregano, thyme, garlic powder, onion powder, red pepper flakes, and salt. Season generously with pepper. Stir well to combine.

5. Add the eggs and use your hands to mix, ensuring everything is coated with egg. Transfer to the prepared baking sheet, and spread it into a thin circle (the thinner the better). Bake for 20 minutes or until the pizza crust is golden brown and crisp around the edges.

6. Brush with pizza sauce and top with mozzarella and the pepperoni. Bake for 10 minutes more or until the cheese melts. Refrigerate leftovers in an airtight container for up to 1 week.

PER SERVING (¼ pizza):
Calories: 521; Total carbs: 10g;
Net carbs: 6g, 8%; Total fat: 40g, 69%;
Protein: 30g, 23%; Fiber: 4g;
Sugar: 5g

VARIATION 1: Calories: 554;
Total carbs: 12g; **Net carbs: 7g, 8%;**
Total fat: 43g, 69%; Protein: 32g, 23%;
Fiber: 5g; Sugar: 5g

VARIATION 2: Calories: 571;
Total carbs: 11g; **Net carbs: 7g, 7%;**
Total fat: 45g, 71%; Protein: 31g, 22%;
Fiber: 4g; Sugar: 5g

VARIATION 1 **SUPREME CAULIFLOWER PIZZA:** Add ½ green bell pepper, diced, ¼ cup cooked sausage, and ¼ cup sliced black olives to the pizza.

VARIATION 2 **CAULIFLOWER PIZZA CRUST WITH CREAM CHEESE:** Get some extra fat in the crust by adding ¼ cup cream cheese (or an additional ¼ cup shredded mozzarella) to the mixture.

CAULIFLOWER GRILLED CHEESE

The first part of this recipe makes a delicious cauliflower "bread" you can use for any sandwich. But I have to say, I think its best use is for grilled cheese. This "bread" keeps really well in the refrigerator (3 to 4 days), so I like to make a bunch at a time and keep it handy throughout the week. I always feel better when I have lots of low-carb lunch options ready to go. **MAKES 2 SANDWICHES**

PREP TIME: 10 minutes
COOK TIME: 25 minutes

1 head cauliflower,
roughly chopped

3 eggs

1 shallot, minced

1 teaspoon dried oregano

1 teaspoon chopped fresh chives

1 teaspoon dried parsley

3 garlic cloves, chopped

1 teaspoon salt, plus more for
seasoning

Freshly ground black pepper

2 tablespoons butter

2 slices Cheddar cheese

1. Preheat the oven to 350°F.

2. Line a baking sheet with parchment paper. Set aside.

3. In a food processor, pulse the cauliflower until roughly chopped (don't overprocess—you want it to be rough). Transfer to a microwave-safe bowl and microwave, uncovered, on high power for 2 minutes. Cool slightly. Place the cauliflower in a thin cloth or piece of cheesecloth and twist to remove any water (not a lot will come out but the little that's there needs to be removed). Transfer to a medium bowl.

4. In a small bowl, whisk together the eggs, shallot, oregano, chives, parsley, garlic, and salt. Season with pepper. Pour the egg mixture over the cauliflower and mix until well incorporated. Scoop the mixture into 4 equal portions on the prepared baking sheet. Spread them out until they're about ¼ inch thick, leaving a little room between each. Bake for 10 minutes, flip, and bake for 7 minutes more. Remove from the oven and cool. Refrigerate in an airtight container for up to 4 days. To reheat, broil quickly in the oven or a toaster oven.

5. Make the sandwiches: in a large nonstick skillet over medium heat, melt 1 tablespoon of butter.

PER SERVING (1 sandwich):
Calories: 440; Total carbs: 27g;
Net carbs: 16g, 22%; Total fat: 29g, 58%;
Protein: 25g, 20%; Fiber: 11g; Sugar: 11g

VARIATION 1: Calories: 540;
Total carbs: 27g; **Net carbs: 16g, 18%;**
Total fat: 34g, 55%; Protein: 38g, 27%;
Fiber: 11g; Sugar: 11g

VARIATION 2: Calories: 614;
Total carbs: 33g; **Net carbs: 17g, 19%;**
Total fat: 43g, 61%; Protein: 20g, 33%;
Fiber: 16g; Sugar: 13g

6. Add 2 pieces of cauliflower bread. Cook for 2 to 3 minutes or until golden brown. Add the remaining 1 tablespoon of butter to the sides facing up then flip the slices. Season with salt and pepper.

7. Add 1 slice of cheese to each piece of bread and let it melt slightly before closing the sandwich. Cook for 1 minute more on each side and serve. Repeat to make the second sandwich.

VARIATION 1 **HAM AND CHEESE MELT ON CAULIFLOWER BREAD:** Add 2 slices deli ham to each sandwich. Follow the rest of the recipe as written.

VARIATION 2 **GRILLED CHEESE WITH BACON AND AVOCADO:** Add 2 slices cooked bacon and ¼ avocado, sliced, to each sandwich.

MAKE AHEAD: Make the cauliflower bread ahead of time and keep it refrigerated so you can make sandwiches any time.

CHEESY CAULIFLOWER GRATIN

This recipe is a keto take on scalloped potatoes, or really any cheesy baked potato dish. I use cauliflower instead of potatoes, but the result is just as good—warm and cheesy baked goodness that's perfect on a chilly evening with a glass of dry red wine. Yum! **MAKES 4 SERVINGS**

PREP TIME: 10 minutes
COOK TIME: 30 minutes

1 head cauliflower, cut into florets

2 tablespoons butter

2 garlic cloves

2 cups heavy (whipping) cream

¼ cup cream cheese

Salt

Freshly ground black pepper

½ cup grated white Cheddar cheese

PER SERVING: Calories: 622; Total carbs: 16g; **Net carbs: 11g, 10%; Total fat: 60g, 84%; Protein: 11g, 6%;** Fiber: 5g; Sugar: 6g

VARIATION 1: Calories: 622; Total carbs: 16g; **Net carbs: 11g, 10%; Total fat: 60g, 84%; Protein: 11g, 6%;** Fiber: 5g; Sugar: 6g

VARIATION 2: Calories: 629; Total carbs: 15g; **Net carbs: 10g, 9%; Total fat: 59g, 83%; Protein: 14g, 8%;** Fiber: 5g; Sugar: 5g

1. Preheat the oven to 400°F.

2. Bring a large saucepan of water to a boil over high heat and add the cauliflower. Boil for 2 to 3 minutes and drain. Transfer the cauliflower to an 8-by-8-inch baking dish.

3. Return the pan to medium heat and add the butter to melt.

4. Add the garlic. Cook for about 2 minutes until fragrant. Reduce the heat to low and, while stirring, add the cream. Simmer for about 2 minutes.

5. Add the cream cheese. Season with salt and pepper. Stir until smooth. Pour the sauce over the cauliflower and top with the Cheddar. Bake for about 20 minutes or until the cheese melts and is golden brown. Refrigerate leftovers in an airtight container for up to 4 days.

VARIATION 1 **SPICY CHEESY CAULIFLOWER GRATIN:** Use pepper jack instead of Cheddar for a spicy kick.

VARIATION 2 **OVEN-BAKED CAULIFLOWER GRATIN:** Save a bit of time by skipping the stove top: Using an 8-by-8-inch baking dish, pour in the cream and sprinkle the garlic over the raw cauliflower florets. Season with salt and pepper. Skip the cream cheese and double up on the white Cheddar. Bake at 375°F for 25 to 30 minutes or until the cheese has melted and the cauliflower is fork-tender.

MASHED CAULIFLOWER

This mashed cauliflower really is as good as real mashed potatoes, and, I swear, some people won't even notice you've made a low-carb switch! The trick is to use enough butter and cream. It's particularly good as a side with steak and a salad. Such an easy, classic dinner that won't throw off your macros one bit. **MAKES 4 SERVINGS**

PREP TIME: 10 minutes
COOK TIME: 15 minutes

8 cups water

1 head cauliflower, washed and chopped

2 to 3 tablespoons butter

1 garlic clove, minced

¼ cup heavy (whipping) cream, plus more as needed

Salt

Freshly ground black pepper

PER SERVING: Calories: 180; Total carbs: 12g; **Net carbs: 7g, 24%; Total fat: 14g, 69%; Protein: 5g, 7%;** Fiber: 5g; Sugar: 5g

VARIATION 1: Calories: 207; Total carbs: 12g; **Net carbs: 7g, 21%; Total fat: 16g, 68%; Protein: 7g, 11%;** Fiber: 5g; Sugar: 5g

VARIATION 2: Calories: 299; Total carbs: 12g; **Net carbs: 7g, 15%; Total fat: 24g, 70%; Protein: 13g, 15%;** Fiber: 5g; Sugar: 5g

1. In a large saucepan over high heat, bring the water to a boil.

2. Add the cauliflower and cook for about 10 minutes or until fork-tender. Remove from the heat, drain, and set aside.

3. Return the pan to medium heat and add the butter and garlic. Sauté for 2 to 3 minutes until the garlic browns slightly.

4. Return the cauliflower to the pan. Use an immersion blender to purée the mixture. If you don't have an immersion blender, carefully transfer everything to a regular blender and purée.

5. Add the cream. Continue to blend until the mashed cauliflower is as smooth as you like it. Season with salt and pepper. If necessary, add another splash of cream (or some chicken broth) to thin it a bit. Serve immediately, or keep warm until ready to serve. Refrigerate leftovers in an airtight container for up to 5 days.

VARIATION 1 **OVEN-BAKED PARMESAN MASHED CAULIFLOWER:** Follow the recipe as written then transfer the mashed cauliflower to a 7-by-11-inch baking dish. Top with ¼ cup grated Parmesan and broil for 3 to 4 minutes or until the cheese turns golden brown.

VARIATION 2 **LOADED MASHED CAULIFLOWER:** Follow the recipe as written and add ½ cup shredded Cheddar, ¼ cup crumbled cooked bacon, and ¼ cup sliced scallion to the mashed cauliflower. Stir gently to combine, and top each serving with a dollop of sour cream.

ALLERGEN TIP: Use coconut cream instead of heavy cream if you don't tolerate lactose.

CURRIED COCONUT CAULIFLOWER

This is a comforting dish that comes together in just one pan and takes fewer than 30 minutes—what more could you want? I love cauliflower with some curry and coconut milk—the flavors blend beautifully together. This is a great recipe year-round. **MAKES 4 SERVINGS**

PREP TIME: 10 minutes
COOK TIME: 20 minutes

1 tablespoon ghee

½ onion, diced

2 garlic cloves

½ serrano chile pepper, seeded and finely diced

1 head cauliflower, washed and trimmed into florets

Salt

Freshly ground black pepper

1 (13.5-ounce) can full-fat coconut milk

3 tablespoons curry powder

PER SERVING: Calories: 310; Total carbs: 15g; **Net carbs: 10g, 17%; Total fat: 28g, 77%; Protein: 6g, 6%;** Fiber: 5g; Sugar: 4g

VARIATION 1: Calories: 444; Total carbs: 15g; **Net carbs: 10g, 12%; Total fat: 33g, 63%; Protein: 28g, 25%;** Fiber: 5g; Sugar: 4g

VARIATION 2: Calories: 311; Total carbs: 15g; **Net carbs: 10g, 17%; Total fat: 28g, 77%; Protein: 6g, 6%;** Fiber: 5g; Sugar: 4g

1. In a large skillet over medium heat, melt the ghee.

2. Add the onion and garlic. Sauté for 5 to 7 minutes until the onion is softened and translucent.

3. Add the serrano and cauliflower. Cook for 4 to 5 minutes more. Season with salt and pepper.

4. Pour the coconut milk over the cauliflower and add the curry powder. Stir to combine. Simmer for 5 minutes to allow the flavors to combine. Serve hot. Refrigerate leftovers in an airtight container for up to 1 week.

VARIATION 1 **CURRIED COCONUT CAULIFLOWER AND CHICKEN:** Make this a main course by adding 1 pound chicken thighs, diced, to the skillet after the garlic and onion. Cook for 5 to 7 minutes or until the chicken starts to brown. Follow the rest of the recipe as written.

VARIATION 2 **CURRIED COCONUT CAULIFLOWER AND ZUCCHINI NOODLES:** Add 2 spiralized zucchini to the pan after the cauliflower and curry powder. Season well with salt and pepper.

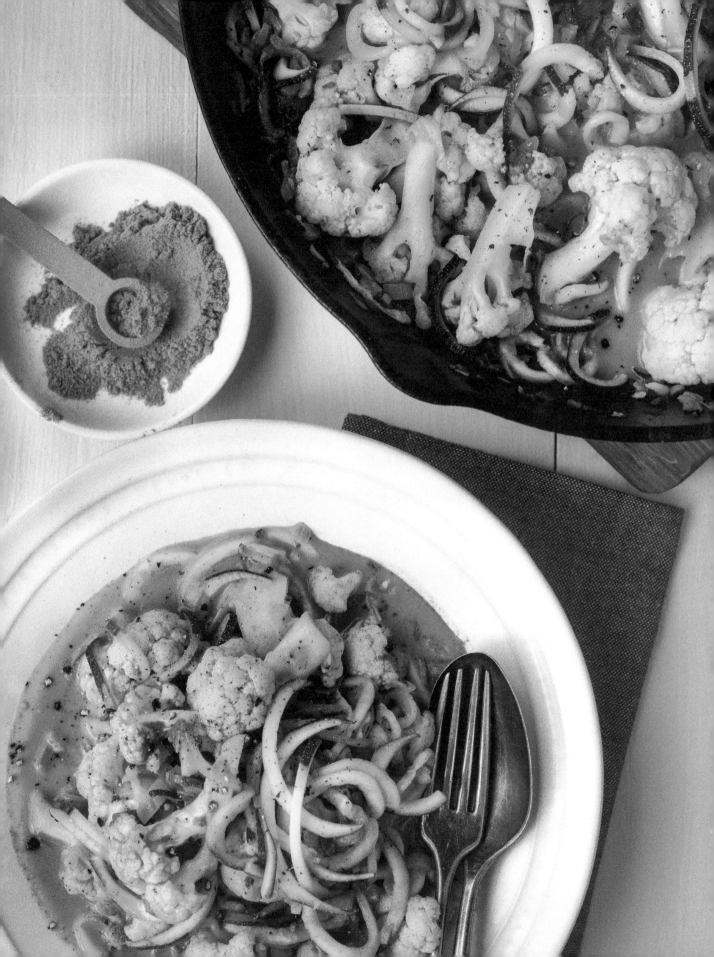

CAULIFLOWER FRITTERS

These fritters are a bit like potato latkes, except they cook slightly faster and they're low-carb because they're made with cauliflower. This is a more keto-friendly recipe that I've adapted from my first book, *The Big 15 Paleo Cookbook*, by adding some mozzarella, which makes these tastier. A little cheese always helps. **MAKES 4 SERVINGS**

PREP TIME: 5 minutes
COOK TIME: 15 minutes

 GF

1 large head cauliflower, chopped into florets

1 or 2 garlic cloves, chopped

¼ cup almond flour

¼ cup shredded mozzarella cheese

2 eggs, whisked

Salt

Freshly ground black pepper

2 tablespoons butter

2 tablespoons sliced scallion, green parts only

PER SERVING: Calories: 170; Total carbs: 12g; **Net carbs: 7g, 27%; Total fat: 11g, 55%; Protein: 9g, 18%;** Fiber: 5g; Sugar: 5g

VARIATION 1: Calories: 228; Total carbs: 16g; **Net carbs: 11g, 26%; Total fat: 16g, 60%; Protein: 10g, 14%;** Fiber: 5g; Sugar: 6g

VARIATION 2: Calories: 170; Total carbs: 11g; **Net carbs: 7g, 24%; Total fat: 11g, 57%; Protein: 10g, 19%;** Fiber: 4g; Sugar: 3g

1. In a large saucepan of boiling water, quickly cook the cauliflower for 5 to 6 minutes or until just fork-tender. Drain and cool slightly. Transfer to a food processor and process until it almost has the consistency of mashed potato. Transfer to a large bowl.

2. Add the garlic, almond flour, mozzarella, and eggs. Season with salt and pepper. Stir until well incorporated.

3. In a large skillet over medium-high heat, melt the butter. Spoon about 2 heaping tablespoons of the cauliflower mixture into your hand and create a patty about half the size of your palm. Repeat with the remaining mixture. Carefully add the patties to the butter (you may have to do this in batches). Cook for about 3 minutes until browned. Flip and cook the other side for about 3 minutes until browned. Serve garnished with the sliced scallion. Refrigerate leftovers in an airtight container for up to 1 week.

VARIATION 1 **CAULIFLOWER FRITTERS WITH GARLIC AIOLI:** Serve these with a side of garlic aioli (see Keto Fish Cakes with Garlic Aioli, page 126).

VARIATION 2 **BROCCOLI FRITTERS:** Use broccoli instead of cauliflower for a green variation.

CAULIFLOWER "TATER" TOTS

Is it just me or are tater tots having a moment? It all started for me a few years ago when I realized one of my favorite hipster sushi bars (that's a thing, you know) served buckets of tots as an appetizer. And then again recently when I became aware of "tachos"—nachos made with tots instead of tortilla chips. The grain-free eater in me was super excited, but to stay low-carb I make these tots with cauliflower instead of potatoes. **MAKES 4 SERVINGS**

PREP TIME: 10 minutes
COOK TIME: 30 minutes

Butter, or olive oil, for the baking sheet

1 head cauliflower, cut into florets

1 egg, whisked

½ onion, minced

½ cup shredded mozzarella cheese

¼ cup grated Parmesan cheese

¼ cup almond flour

Salt

Freshly ground black pepper

PER SERVING: Calories: 136; Total carbs: 9g; **Net carbs: 5g, 26%; Total fat: 7g, 46%; Protein: 10g, 28%;** Fiber: 4g; Sugar: 4g

VARIATION 1: Calories: 202; Total carbs: 10g; **Net carbs: 6g, 17%; Total fat: 12g, 55%; Protein: 15g, 28%;** Fiber: 4g; Sugar: 5g

VARIATION 2: Calories: 226; Total carbs: 9g; **Net carbs: 5g, 15%; Total fat: 17g, 68%; Protein: 10g, 17%;** Fiber: 4g; Sugar: 4g

1. Preheat the oven to 375°F.

2. Lightly grease a baking sheet with butter. Set aside.

3. In a large saucepan, cook the cauliflower in boiling water for 2 to 3 minutes or until softened. Transfer to a food processor and pulse until fine. Transfer to a large bowl.

4. Add the egg, onion, mozzarella, Parmesan, and almond flour. Season with salt and pepper and mix well to combine. Spoon about 1 tablespoon at a time into your hand and mold it into traditional tot shape (small rounded rectangles). Place on the prepared baking sheet and bake for 20 to 25 minutes or until golden brown.

VARIATION 1 **KETO "TACHOS:"** Arrange hot tots on a platter and top with ½ cup shredded Cheddar, ¼ cup Low-Carb Chili (page 98), and some sliced scallion.

VARIATION 2 **FRIED CAULIFLOWER "TATER" TOTS:** If you have a little more time, panfry the tots in a large nonstick skillet over medium-high heat in 2 to 3 tablespoons olive oil or ghee for 2 to 3 minutes per side or until crispy and browned.

CAULIFLOWER CHEESY GARLIC BREAD

This recipe is similar to Cauliflower Pizza (page 166), but instead of Italian spices I add more garlic powder and lots of cheese to create a delicious cheesy bread. This makes an awesome after-school snack for your kids and their friends, or a tasty appetizer for dinner and a movie at home on a weekend. I just love cauliflower and mozzarella together with a little marinara or tomato sauce—it really does hit all the same flavor spots that pizza does, and what's better than pizza? **MAKES 6 SERVINGS**

PREP TIME: 10 minutes
COOK TIME: 30 minutes

Butter, or olive oil, for the baking sheet

1 head cauliflower, roughly chopped into florets

3 cups shredded mozzarella cheese, divided

½ cup grated Parmesan cheese

¼ cup cream cheese, at room temperature

3 teaspoons garlic powder, plus more for sprinkling

1 teaspoon onion powder

½ teaspoon red pepper flakes

1 tablespoon salt, plus more for seasoning

Freshly ground black pepper

2 eggs, whisked

Sugar-free marinara sauce, warmed, for dipping

1. Preheat the oven to 400°F.

2. Grease a baking sheet with butter. Set aside. Alternatively, use a pizza stone.

3. In a food processor, pulse the cauliflower until fine. Transfer to a microwave-safe bowl and microwave on high power, uncovered, for 2 minutes. Cool slightly. Place the cauliflower in a thin cloth or piece of cheesecloth and twist to remove any water (not a lot will come out but the little that's there needs to be removed). Transfer to a large bowl.

4. Add 2 cups of mozzarella, the Parmesan, cream cheese, garlic powder, onion powder, red pepper flakes, and salt. Season generously with black pepper. Stir well to combine.

5. Add the eggs and use your hands to mix, ensuring everything is coated with egg. Transfer to the prepared baking sheet. Spread the mixture out into a large rectangle, about 1 inch thick. Sprinkle with more salt, pepper, and garlic powder. Bake for 20 minutes or until the bread starts to turn golden brown.

6. Remove from the oven, top with the remaining 1 cup of mozzarella, and bake for about 10 minutes more or until the cheese melts. Cool slightly and cut into breadsticks. Serve with the marinara sauce for dipping. Refrigerate leftovers in an airtight container for up to 4 days.

PER SERVING: Calories: 296;
Total carbs: 10g; **Net carbs: 7g, 12%;**
Total fat: 20g, 60%; Protein: 21g, 28%;
Fiber: 3g; Sugar: 5g

VARIATION 1: Calories: 296;
Total carbs: 10g; **Net carbs: 7g, 12%;**
Total fat: 20g, 60%; Protein: 21g, 28%;
Fiber: 3g; Sugar: 5g

VARIATION 2: Calories: 527;
Total carbs: 10g; **Net carbs: 7g, 7%;**
Total fat: 41g, 69%; Protein: 31g, 24%;
Fiber: 3g; Sugar: 5g

VARIATION 1 **HERBY CAULIFLOWER CHEESY GARLIC BREAD:**
Add 1 tablespoon chopped fresh rosemary leaves and 1 tablespoon chopped fresh oregano leaves to the cauliflower mix. Follow the rest of the recipe as written.

VARIATION 2 **CHEESY CAULIFLOWER PIZZA BREAD:** Add 8 to 10 ounces chopped pepperoni to the mix.

CAULIFLOWER RICE

This is a very basic cauliflower rice recipe that is great with some butter on it as a side with any beef, chicken, pork, or seafood recipe in this book. You can also add different seasonings and make an Asian-style fried rice or a great cheesy rice dish (see both variations). **MAKES 4 SERVINGS**

PREP TIME: 15 minutes
COOK TIME: 15 minutes

1 head cauliflower, washed and cut into rough chunks

2 tablespoons olive oil

Salt

Freshly ground black pepper

PER SERVING: Calories: 112; Total carbs: 11g; **Net carbs: 6g, 36%; Total fat: 7g, 55%; Protein: 4g, 9%;** Fiber: 5g; Sugar: 5g

VARIATION 1: Calories: 169; Total carbs: 13g; **Net carbs: 7g, 29%; Total fat: 12g, 63%; Protein: 5g, 8%;** Fiber: 6g; Sugar: 6g

VARIATION 2: Calories: 169; Total carbs: 11g; **Net carbs: 6g, 24%; Total fat: 12g, 61%; Protein: 8g, 15%;** Fiber: 5g; Sugar: 5g

1. In a food processor, pulse the cauliflower for 2 to 3 minutes until it resembles the texture of regular rice. Transfer to a large nonstick pan over medium heat and cook for 5 to 7 minutes, stirring occasionally. (Do this without any fat first so you can dry the cauliflower a bit, which will help it get crispy later.)

2. Add the olive oil and increase the heat to medium high. Cook for 5 to 7 minutes more or until the cauliflower turns golden brown and is slightly crispy. Season with salt and pepper and serve. Refrigerate leftovers in an airtight container for up to 3 days. Reheat in a skillet over medium-high heat.

VARIATION 1 **ASIAN CAULIFLOWER FRIED RICE:** Add 1½ tablespoons sesame oil, 1 diced carrot, 2 tablespoons peas, ¼ teaspoon grated fresh ginger, and ¼ teaspoon red pepper flakes. Stir well and add 2 tablespoons soy sauce. Move the rice over to the side of the skillet. Crack 1 egg into the pan and stir to scramble it. Combine the egg with the rice and serve hot.

VARIATION 2 **CHEESY CAULIFLOWER RICE:** Add ½ cup shredded cheese to the cauliflower rice before serving. Stir well and let melt.

ROASTED BUFFALO CAULIFLOWER

This is a recipe I started making about four years ago—I had a head of cauliflower and no plans for it, but my husband and I are really into buffalo sauce, so I thought I'd roast the cauliflower and toss it in some buffalo! The result was perfect, and I actually make it more as an appetizer now than I do a side dish (although it is great as a side with virtually any protein or salad).

MAKES 4 SERVINGS

PREP TIME: 10 minutes
COOK TIME: 30 to 40 minutes

1 head cauliflower, washed and chopped into florets

2 tablespoons olive oil

Salt

Freshly ground black pepper

4 tablespoons butter

¼ cup Frank's RedHot Sauce

Sliced scallion, green parts only, for garnish

PER SERVING: Calories: 214;
Total carbs: 11g; **Net carbs: 6g, 19%;**
Total fat: 18g, 76%; Protein: 4g, 5%;
Fiber: 5g; Sugar: 5g

VARIATION 1: Calories: 213;
Total carbs: 10g; **Net carbs: 6g, 18%;**
Total fat: 19g, 77%; Protein: 5g, 5%;
Fiber: 4g; Sugar: 3g

VARIATION 2: Calories: 400;
Total carbs: 12g; **Net carbs: 7g, 10%;**
Total fat: 29g, 63%; Protein: 27g, 27%;
Fiber: 5g; Sugar: 5g

1. Preheat the oven to 400°F.

2. Place the cauliflower on a baking sheet, drizzle with the olive oil, and season with salt and pepper. Bake for 30 to 40 minutes or until golden brown.

3. While the cauliflower roasts, in a small saucepan over medium heat, melt the butter and hot sauce together. Stir until combined and smooth with no lumps.

4. Remove the cauliflower from the oven and transfer to a large bowl. Pour the sauce over and toss well to combine. Serve immediately, garnished with scallion.

VARIATION 1 **ROASTED BUFFALO BROCCOLI:** Use broccoli instead of cauliflower.

VARIATION 2 **ROASTED BUFFALO CHICKEN AND CAULIFLOWER:** Make this a main course by adding 1 pound diced boneless skinless chicken thighs to the roasting pan with the cauliflower. (You might want to make another half batch of buffalo sauce.)

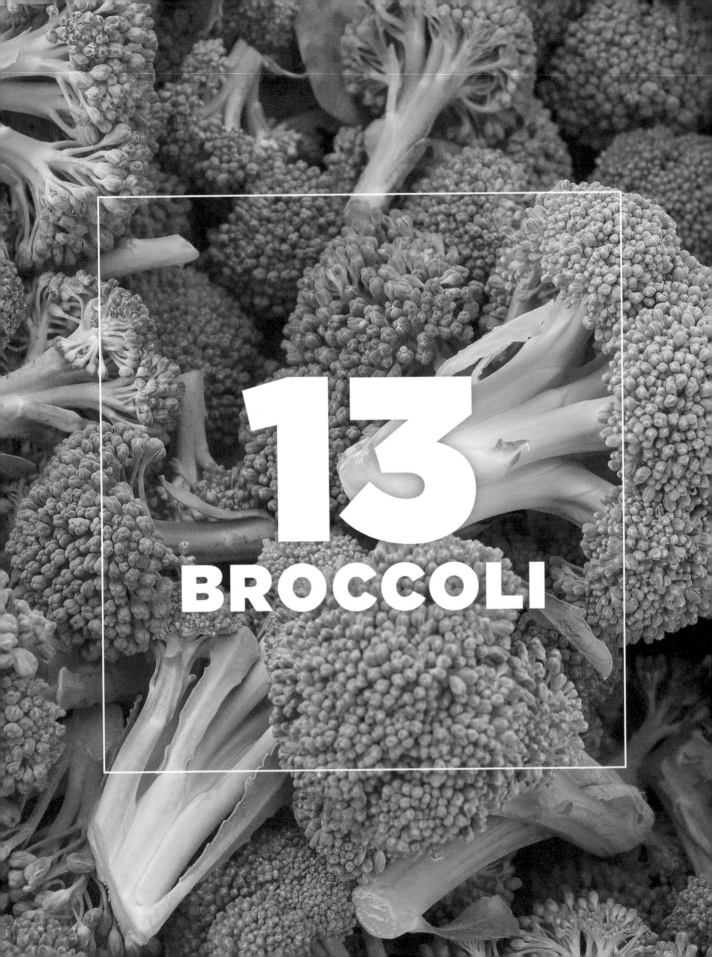

13
BROCCOLI

Broccoli is one of those vegetables that often gets overlooked because people think it's boring. Truth is, it has great flavor and texture and you can do so many creative and flavorful things with it! In this chapter we'll make casseroles, soups, salads, and even noodles with broccoli—save your stalks, we can spiralize those! (There's actually a whole broccoli chapter in my second cookbook, *The Big 10 Paleo Spiralizer Cookbook*, which is dedicated entirely to making noodles out of veggies.)

Broccoli is a great keto veggie option because you can cook it multiple ways and it's delicious paired with dairy—cream, cream cheese, shredded cheese, it's all good. I hope some of these recipes inspire you to pick up a few heads of broccoli the next time you're picking out veggies at the market.

SAVORY BROCCOLI CHEDDAR WAFFLES

These waffles are sure to be a hit at your next brunch party. The recipe is somewhat similar to the cauliflower bread you make for Cauliflower Grilled Cheese (page 168), but here we use broccoli and cook it in a waffle iron instead of the oven! So you don't need to worry about missing waffles and pancakes; these veggie-packed replacements fit into the keto diet just fine.

MAKES 4 SERVINGS

PREP TIME: 15 minutes
COOK TIME: 20 minutes

1 head broccoli, florets separated, stalk reserved for another use

1 shallot, minced

3 eggs

1 teaspoon chopped fresh chives

3 garlic cloves, minced

1 teaspoon salt

Freshly ground black pepper

1 cup shredded Cheddar cheese

Nonstick olive oil cooking spray, or olive oil, for the waffle iron

Sliced scallion, for garnish

PER SERVING: Calories: 224; Total carbs: 12g; **Net carbs: 8g, 19%; Total fat: 14g, 54%; Protein: 16g, 27%;** Fiber: 4g; Sugar: 3g

VARIATION 1: Calories: 334; Total carbs: 12g; **Net carbs: 8g, 14%; Total fat: 23g, 60%; Protein: 23g, 26%;** Fiber: 4g; Sugar: 3g

VARIATION 2: Calories: 316; Total carbs: 18g; **Net carbs: 10g, 20%; Total fat: 21g, 60%; Protein: 18g, 20%;** Fiber: 8g; Sugar: 5g

1. In a food processor, pulse the broccoli florets until roughly chopped (don't overprocess—you want it to be rough). Transfer to a microwave-safe container and microwave, uncovered, on high power for 2 minutes. Cool slightly. Place the broccoli in a thin cloth or piece of cheesecloth and twist to remove any water (not a lot will come out but the little that's there needs to be removed). Transfer to a medium bowl and add the shallot. Stir to combine.

2. In a small bowl, whisk together the eggs, chives, garlic, and salt, and season with pepper. Pour the egg mixture over the broccoli and mix together until well incorporated.

3. Add the Cheddar and continue to mix gently.

4. Turn on your waffle iron. Grease it well with cooking spray (if you don't have cooking spray, use a little olive oil on a paper towel).

5. Separate the broccoli mixture into 4 portions. Spoon the mixture onto the prepared waffle iron. Cook for 4 to 5 minutes (or follow the manufacturer's instructions if you're unsure) or until the waffle "batter" is firm and golden brown. Top with sliced scallion and serve.

LOADED BROCCOLI CHEDDAR WAFFLES:
Top these waffles with crumbled cooked bacon, more Cheddar, and a dollop of sour cream.

BROCCOLI PEPPER JACK WAFFLES WITH AVOCADO: Use pepper jack instead of Cheddar and serve with smashed avocado on top.

MAKE AHEAD TIP: You can make the "batter" the night before and store it in an airtight container in the fridge so you're ready to cook in the morning.

CHEESY BROCCOLI CASSEROLE

This casserole is a great vegetarian option that's also filling, so you won't ever feel like it's not hearty enough to be a main course. I love the combination of broccoli with Cheddar (obviously), but the cream cheese really kicks it up a notch. Put this on your list for your next Meatless Monday—I bet you'll love it.

MAKES 4 SERVINGS

PREP TIME: 10 minutes
COOK TIME: 35 minutes

2 tablespoons butter

¼ white onion, diced

1 garlic clove, minced

1 pound broccoli florets, roughly chopped

Salt

Freshly ground black pepper

4 ounces cream cheese, at room temperature

1 cup shredded Cheddar cheese, divided

½ cup heavy (whipping) cream

2 eggs

PER SERVING: Calories: 440; Total carbs: 11g; **Net carbs: 8g, 9%;** **Total fat: 39g, 77%; Protein: 16g, 14%;** Fiber: 3g; Sugar: 3g

VARIATION 1: Calories: 466; Total carbs: 11g; **Net carbs: 8g, 9%;** **Total fat: 41g, 77%; Protein: 17g, 14%;** Fiber: 3g; Sugar: 4g

VARIATION 2: Calories: 657; Total carbs: 11g; **Net carbs: 8g, 6%;** **Total fat: 53g, 71%; Protein: 38g, 23%;** Fiber: 3g; Sugar: 3g

1. Preheat the oven to 350°F.

2. In a large skillet over medium heat, melt the butter.

3. Add the onion and garlic. Sauté for 5 to 7 minutes until the onion is softened and translucent.

4. Add the broccoli. Season with salt and pepper. Cook for 4 to 5 minutes until just softened. Transfer to a 7-by-11-inch baking dish.

5. In a medium bowl, stir together the cream cheese, ½ cup of Cheddar, the cream, and eggs. Pour over the broccoli. Season with more salt and pepper, and top with the remaining ½ cup of Cheddar. Bake for 20 minutes. Refrigerate leftovers in an airtight container for up to 1 week.

VARIATION 1 **BUFFALO BLUE CHEESE BROCCOLI CASSEROLE:** Add ½ cup Frank's RedHot Sauce and an additional 2 tablespoons melted butter to the casserole dish. Stir well to combine. Follow the rest of the recipe as written and serve topped with ½ cup crumbled blue cheese and some sliced scallion.

VARIATION 2 **CHEESY BROCCOLI CASSEROLE WITH BEEF:** Add 1 pound ground beef to the pan before you cook the broccoli. Follow the rest of the recipe as written.

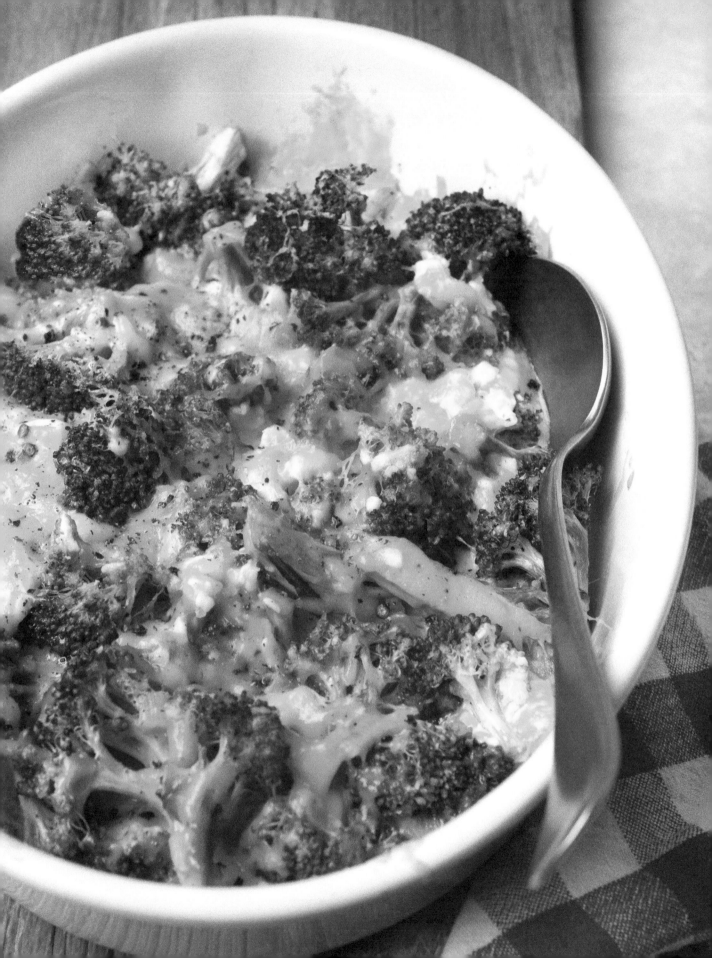

BROCCOLI CHEDDAR SOUP

A lot of soups like this one usually start with some butter and flour to thicken it up, but I've found that if you skip the flour it really doesn't make a difference, especially if you use heavy cream instead of regular milk. This soup is warm and nourishing and, more importantly, keto-friendly. **MAKES 4 SERVINGS**

PREP TIME: 10 minutes
COOK TIME: 15 minutes

4 tablespoons butter

1 celery stalk, diced

1 carrot, diced

½ onion, diced

1 garlic clove, minced

3 cups chicken broth

2 cups broccoli florets

1 cup heavy (whipping) cream

2 ½ cups shredded
Cheddar cheese

Salt

Freshly ground black pepper

PER SERVING: Calories: 638;
Total carbs: 10g; **Net carbs: 8g, 5%;**
Total fat: 58g, 80%; Protein: 23g, 15%;
Fiber: 2g; Sugar: 3g

VARIATION 1: Calories: 721;
Total carbs: 10g; **Net carbs: 8g, 5%;**
Total fat: 64g, 78%; Protein: 29g, 17%;
Fiber: 2g; Sugar: 3g

VARIATION 2: Calories: 856;
Total carbs: 10g; **Net carbs: 8g, 5%;**
Total fat: 72g, 74%; Protein: 45g, 21%;
Fiber: 2g; Sugar: 3g

1. In a large saucepan over medium heat, melt the butter.

2. Add the celery, carrot, onion, and garlic. Stir to combine and sauté for 5 to 7 minutes until softened.

3. Stir in the chicken broth and bring to a simmer.

4. Add the broccoli. Simmer for 5 to 7 minutes then add the cream.

5. While stirring, slowly add the Cheddar, letting it melt completely. Season well with salt and pepper and serve hot. Refrigerate leftovers in an airtight container for up to 1 week.

VARIATION 1 **BACON BROCCOLI CHEDDAR SOUP:** Top each serving with 2 pieces crumbled cooked bacon.

VARIATION 2 **CHEESEBURGER BROCCOLI SOUP:** Add 1 pound ground beef to the saucepan after the butter, celery, carrot, onion, and garlic. Cook for 7 to 10 minutes or until browned. Follow the rest of the recipe as written.

PERFECT PAIR: Serve as a side with The Classic Juicy Lucy (page 102) or Keto Meatloaf (page 104).

COCONUT CURRY BROCCOLI SOUP

This soup is a nice departure from broccoli soups that usually contain a lot of dairy—the creaminess here comes from coconut milk. So, nondairy eaters, you can enjoy this without having to make any substitutions! This version is a little spicy, but you can definitely add more red pepper flakes (or even a fresh diced chile pepper) to add some extra heat if you like your curry hotter.

MAKES 4 SERVINGS

PREP TIME: 10 minutes
COOK TIME: 20 minutes

4 tablespoons butter

1 celery stalk, diced

1 carrot, diced

½ onion, diced

1 garlic clove, minced

2 tablespoons curry powder

1 teaspoon red pepper flakes

3 cups chicken broth

2 cups broccoli florets

1 cup canned coconut cream

Salt

Freshly ground black pepper

PER SERVING: Calories: 274; Total carbs: 11g; **Net carbs: 8g, 13%;** **Total fat: 25g, 78%; Protein: 7g, 9%;** Fiber: 3g; Sugar: 3g

VARIATION 1: Calories: 409; Total carbs: 11g; **Net carbs: 8g, 9%;** **Total fat: 29g, 62%; Protein: 29g, 29%;** Fiber: 3g; Sugar: 3g

VARIATION 2: Calories: 271; Total carbs: 10g; **Net carbs: 7g, 12%;** **Total fat: 25g, 79%; Protein: 6g, 9%;** Fiber: 3g; Sugar: 3g

1. In a large saucepan over medium heat, melt the butter.

2. Add the celery, carrot, onion, garlic, curry powder, and red pepper flakes. Stir to combine. Sauté for 5 to 7 minutes until the vegetables soften.

3. Stir in the chicken broth and bring to a simmer.

4. Add the broccoli and simmer for 5 to 7 minutes.

5. Stir in the coconut cream and simmer for 5 to 10 minutes more until the broccoli is cooked. Season well with salt and pepper and serve hot. Refrigerate leftovers in an airtight container for up to 1 week.

VARIATION 1 **CHICKEN COCONUT CURRY BROCCOLI SOUP:** Add some protein. Add 1 pound chicken thighs, diced, to the simmering chicken broth, where they'll slowly cook.

VARIATION 2 **COCONUT CURRY CAULIFLOWER SOUP:** Swap out the broccoli for cauliflower if you've got it.

ROASTED LEMON GARLIC BROCCOLI

This is a huge hit every time I make it. The trick is to slice the broccoli florets thinly so they have plenty of surface area to get nice and crispy. Olive oil and high heat are a great combination for roasting hearty green veggies such as broccoli and Brussels sprouts—I make a big batch of veggies like this at least once a week. **MAKES 4 SERVINGS**

PREP TIME: 10 minutes
COOK TIME: 15 minutes

1 large head broccoli, cut into florets and thinly sliced

½ cup olive oil

1 teaspoon garlic powder

1 teaspoon red pepper flakes

Salt

Freshly ground black pepper

Juice of 1 lemon

PER SERVING: Calories: 293; Total carbs: 11g; **Net carbs: 7g, 13%; Total fat: 28g, 83%; Protein: 4g, 4%;** Fiber: 4g; Sugar: 3g

VARIATION 1: Calories: 384; Total carbs: 17g; **Net carbs: 9g, 16%; Total fat: 35g, 80%; Protein: 6g, 4%;** Fiber: 8g; Sugar: 5g

VARIATION 2: Calories: 293; Total carbs: 11g; **Net carbs: 7g, 13%; Total fat: 28g, 83%; Protein: 4g, 4%;** Fiber: 4g; Sugar: 3g

1. Preheat the oven to 400°F.

2. In a large bowl, toss together the broccoli, olive oil, garlic powder, and red pepper flakes. Season with salt and pepper. Transfer to a rimmed baking sheet and bake for 15 to 17 minutes or until the broccoli browns slightly and is crispy around the edges.

3. Squeeze the lemon juice over the broccoli. Stir to combine and serve hot. Refrigerate leftovers in an airtight container for up to 1 week.

VARIATION 1 **ROASTED LEMON GARLIC BROCCOLI WITH AVOCADO:** Serve this broccoli with diced avocado on top—¼ avocado per serving.

VARIATION 2 **PANFRIED LEMON GARLIC BROCCOLI:** If you don't feel like turning on your oven, make this dish in a skillet! Cook for 10 to 15 minutes over medium-high heat, stirring occasionally.

PERFECT PAIR: Serve with Steak and Mushroom Kebabs (page 97).

SPIRALIZED BROCCOLI NOODLES

Did you know you can turn broccoli stalks into noodles? My mind was blown the first time I tried it—I used to throw them away! This recipe is easy and fun: you turn the broccoli stems into noodles and add the florets, sauté everything in some butter and garlic, and end with some Parmesan. It's like a grown-up version of buttery noodles, made completely from vegetables. **MAKES 4 SERVINGS**

PREP TIME: 10 minutes
COOK TIME: 10 minutes

2 tablespoons butter

1 garlic clove, minced

2 heads broccoli, florets removed, stalks spiralized, or peeled with a vegetable peeler into strips and cut into noodles

Salt

Freshly ground black pepper

¼ cup grated Parmesan cheese

PER SERVING: Calories: 104; Total carbs: 6g; **Net carbs: 4g, 20%; Total fat: 8g, 65%; Protein: 5g, 15%;** Fiber: 2g; Sugar: 1g

VARIATION 1: Calories: 336; Total carbs: 7g; **Net carbs: 5g, 9%; Total fat: 32g, 82%; Protein: 8g, 9%;** Fiber: 2g; Sugar: 2g

VARIATION 2: Calories: 166; Total carbs: 6g; **Net carbs: 4g, 13%; Total fat: 12g, 66%; Protein: 9g, 21%;** Fiber: 2g; Sugar: 1g

1. In a medium skillet over medium heat, melt the butter and add the garlic. Cook for 2 to 3 minutes.

2. Add the broccoli florets. Cook for 3 to 4 minutes.

3. Add the broccoli noodles. Cook for 4 to 5 minutes more. Season with salt and pepper and top with the Parmesan. Refrigerate leftovers in an airtight container for up to 1 week.

VARIATION 1 **SPIRALIZED BROCCOLI NOODLES ALFREDO:** Make this veggie noodle dish cream-based by tossing it in ½ cup Alfredo sauce (see Shrimp Alfredo, page 138).

VARIATION 2 **CRISPY PROSCIUTTO SPIRALIZED BROCCOLI NOODLES:** Add 8 ounces chopped prosciutto to the skillet when you sauté the garlic.

PESTO BROCCOLI SALAD

This salad is a tasty way to enjoy raw broccoli. The trick is to cut it into small pieces so you don't feel like you're struggling with chunky pieces that can sometimes be hard to chew. Add a little red onion and some pesto and you've got a really delicious salad or side for your next lunch or dinner. **MAKES 4 SERVINGS**

PREP TIME: 15 minutes
COOK TIME: 0 minutes

1 large head broccoli, cut into bite-size pieces

¼ red onion, finely diced

¾ cup pesto (see Basil Alfredo Sea Bass, page 132)

Salt

Freshly ground black pepper

Freshly grated Parmesan cheese, for topping

PER SERVING: Calories: 251;
Total carbs: 15g; **Net carbs: 10g, 27%;**
Total fat: 18g, 65%; Protein: 7g, 8%;
Fiber: 5g; Sugar: 4g

VARIATION 1: Calories: 334;
Total carbs: 15g; **Net carbs: 10g, 21%;**
Total fat: 24g, 65%; Protein: 13g, 14%;
Fiber: 5g; Sugar: 4g

VARIATION 2: Calories: 259;
Total carbs: 17g; **Net carbs: 12g, 28%;**
Total fat: 18g, 63%; Protein: 7g, 9%;
Fiber: 5g; Sugar: 4g

In a large bowl, toss together the broccoli, red onion, and pesto. Season with salt and pepper. If possible, let it sit for about 20 minutes before serving to allow the dressing to combine fully with the broccoli. Top with Parmesan and enjoy.

VARIATION 1 **BACON PESTO BROCCOLI SALAD:** Add 8 ounces crumbled cooked bacon to the salad.

VARIATION 2 **PESTO KALE AND BROCCOLI SALAD:** Add 1 cup massaged chopped kale (pour 1 teaspoon olive oil over the kale and massage with your fingers for about 5 minutes) to the broccoli salad. You might need to add an additional ¼ cup pesto.

MAKE IT PALEO: Make the pesto without Parmesan and it'll still be super tasty.

LOW-CARB BEEF WITH BROCCOLI

Beef with broccoli is one of my favorite dishes to order at a Chinese restaurant (and by now you know how much I love Chinese food!), but, unfortunately, it's usually full of flour and cornstarch and other carb-laden additives. This one is more on the Paleo side, and definitely keto friendly—just veggies, butter, and steak with some seasonings. I like to make this on a Friday or Saturday night to celebrate the weekend with a nice long Netflix binge and some homemade, low-carb Chinese food! **MAKES 4 SERVINGS**

PREP TIME: 10 minutes
COOK TIME: 20 minutes

1 tablespoon butter

½ onion, diced

2 garlic cloves, minced

1 tablespoon sesame oil

1 pound steak, such as skirt, thinly sliced

1 head broccoli, chopped into florets, florets chopped into bite-size pieces

2 tablespoons gluten-free soy sauce

¼ teaspoon red pepper flakes

2 tablespoons sesame seeds

2 or 3 scallions, green parts only, chopped

PER SERVING: Calories: 514; Total carbs: 14g; **Net carbs: 9g, 10%; Total fat: 41g, 70%; Protein: 26g, 20%;** Fiber: 5g; Sugar: 3g

VARIATION 1: Calories: 529; Total carbs: 16g; **Net carbs: 10g, 11%; Total fat: 41g, 69%; Protein: 28g, 20%;** Fiber: 6g; Sugar: 4g

VARIATION 2: Calories: 493; Total carbs: 10g; **Net carbs: 6g, 7%; Total fat: 41g, 73%; Protein: 24g, 20%;** Fiber: 4g; Sugar: 2g

1. In a large skillet or wok over medium heat, melt the butter.

2. Add the onion and garlic. Sauté for 5 to 7 minutes until the onion is softened and translucent.

3. Add the sesame oil and steak. Cook for 5 to 6 minutes or until the meat begins to brown on all sides.

4. Add the broccoli to the skillet. Cook for 3 to 4 minutes, stirring to combine everything.

5. Add the soy sauce and red pepper flakes. Remove from the heat, transfer to plates, and garnish with the sesame seeds and scallions.

VARIATION 1 **LOW-CARB BEEF WITH BROCCOLI AND MUSHROOMS:** Add 10 ounces sliced mushrooms to the skillet while sautéing the onion and garlic.

VARIATION 2 **LOW-CARB BEEF WITH BROCCOLI AND SUGAR SNAP PEAS:** Use half the amount of broccoli and add ½ cup sugar snap peas to the skillet. Follow the rest of the recipe as written.

MAKE IT PALEO: Use coconut aminos instead of soy sauce in the same amount.

PERFECT PAIR: Serve this dish over a bowl of Cauliflower Rice (page 178).

WARM BACON BROCCOLI SALAD

Spinach and bacon together in a salad, especially when warmed slightly, is so tasty. The addition of broccoli gives this salad a nice crunch—you cook the broccoli only lightly, just so it's warm enough to wilt the spinach. The addition of bacon and red onion and a good red wine vinaigrette makes it the perfect light lunch or salad to go with a dinner entrée. **MAKES 2 SALADS**

PREP TIME: 15 minutes
COOK TIME: 5 minutes

2 cups fresh spinach leaves

¼ cup avocado oil

¼ cup red wine vinegar

1 tablespoon Dijon mustard

½ cup broccoli florets

1 tablespoon olive oil

¼ red onion, thinly sliced

Salt

Freshly ground black pepper

2 or 3 cooked bacon slices, cut widthwise into strips

PER SERVING (1 salad): Calories: 400; Total carbs: 4g; **Net carbs: 2g, 5%;** **Total fat: 40g, 89%; Protein: 6g, 6%;** Fiber: 2g; Sugar: 1g

VARIATION 1: Calories: 499; Total carbs: 6g; **Net carbs: 4g, 6%;** **Total fat: 48g, 85%; Protein: 12g, 9%;** Fiber: 2g; Sugar: 3g

VARIATION 2: Calories: 491; Total carbs: 10g; **Net carbs: 4g, 9%;** **Total fat: 48g, 85%; Protein: 8g, 6%;** Fiber: 6g; Sugar: 3g

1. Place the spinach in a large bowl. Set aside.

2. In a small bowl, whisk the avocado oil, vinegar, and mustard. Set aside.

3. In a large skillet over medium-low heat, gently sauté the broccoli in the olive oil for about 4 minutes. Add the warm broccoli to the spinach, letting the broccoli slightly wilt the spinach leaves.

4. Add the red onion to the skillet. Give the dressing another whisk, add it to the bacon and spinach, and toss everything to coat. Season with salt and pepper. Top with the bacon strips and divide between two salad bowls.

VARIATION 1 **WARM BACON BROCCOLI SALAD WITH FETA:** Add ½ cup crumbled feta cheese to the salad before serving. Toss well to combine.

VARIATION 2 **WARM BACON BROCCOLI SALAD WITH AVOCADO:** Add ½ avocado, diced, to the salad before serving. Toss well to combine.

CHICKEN BROCCOLI ALFREDO

Is there a more classic combination than chicken, broccoli, and Alfredo sauce? This is an easy weeknight dinner recipe that I hope you'll turn to time and again. It all comes together in one pan, which is always a good thing when it comes time to clean up the kitchen! **MAKES 4 SERVINGS**

PREP TIME: 15 minutes
COOK TIME: 15 minutes

1 tablespoon butter

1 garlic clove, minced

1 pound boneless skinless chicken breasts, diced

Salt

Freshly ground black pepper

1 large head broccoli, cut into florets

1½ cups Alfredo sauce (see Basil Alfredo Sea Bass, page 132)

¼ cup grated Parmesan cheese

PER SERVING: Calories: 597; Total carbs: 13g; **Net carbs: 9g, 9%; Total fat: 43g, 63%; Protein: 42g, 28%;** Fiber: 4g; Sugar: 3g

VARIATION 1: Calories: 597; Total carbs: 13g; **Net carbs: 9g, 9%; Total fat: 43g, 63%; Protein: 42g, 28%;** Fiber: 4g; Sugar: 3g

VARIATION 2: Calories: 597; Total carbs: 13g; **Net carbs: 9g, 9%; Total fat: 43g, 63%; Protein: 42g, 28%;** Fiber: 4g; Sugar: 3g

1. Preheat the oven to 350°F.

2. In a large ovenproof skillet over medium heat, melt the butter.

3. Add the garlic. Sauté for about 2 minutes until fragrant.

4. Add the chicken and stir. Season with salt and pepper. Cook for 5 to 7 minutes, stirring, until the chicken begins to brown.

5. Add the broccoli and continue to stir. Cook for 3 to 4 minutes more.

6. Pour the Alfredo sauce over everything, stirring to combine.

7. Top with the Parmesan and transfer to the oven for 5 to 7 minutes or until the cheese browns slightly. Refrigerate leftovers in an airtight container for up to 5 days.

VARIATION 1 **CHICKEN BROCCOLI ALFREDO BAKE:** Skip the stove top. Place the diced chicken breasts in a baking dish with the broccoli. Drizzle with olive oil and season with salt, pepper, and 1 teaspoon garlic powder. Pour the Alfredo sauce over, add the Parmesan, and bake at 350°F for about 25 to 30 minutes or until the chicken is cooked through.

VARIATION 2 **CHICKEN BROCCOLI ALFREDO WITH BROCCOLI NOODLES:** Spiralize the broccoli stalk and add the noodles to the pan with the garlic.

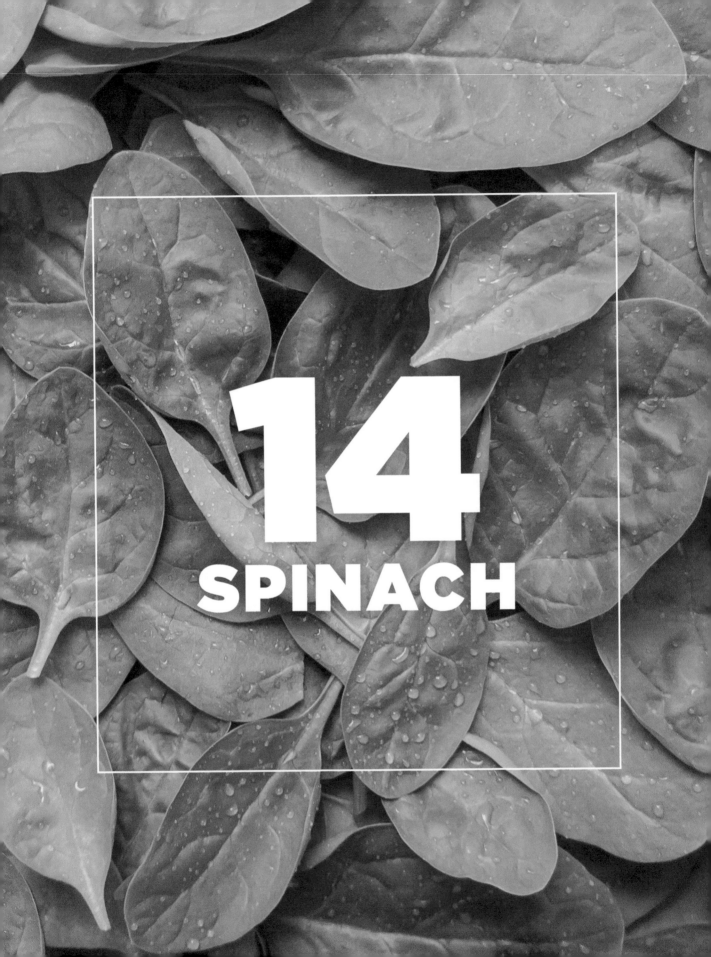

14
SPINACH

I *really* love spinach—I always keep a huge bag of it and, literally, add a handful to every plate before serving. We drizzle Ranch Dressing (page 225) over it for the easiest salad ever. I also like throwing a handful into eggs, smoothies, whatever—it doesn't have a ton of flavor and, if you chop it first, your kids or partner or even you might not notice it's there. These recipes, however, highlight spinach a bit more than that.

Spinach is not only very low in carbs but also has tons of vitamins and minerals: vitamins A, B_2, B_6, and K, manganese, folate, magnesium, iron, calcium, potassium, and so much more. You really get a lot of nutritional bang for your buck, which, again, is why I always keep it around. The following recipes are full of spinach and range from easy breakfasts you can make ahead of time and serve all week to some salads, lunches, dinners, and even snacks! No need to just throw it on a plate all by itself; there are plenty of ways to get spinach into your diet right here.

ZIA'S SPINACH TORTA

This spinach torta is a family recipe from my mom's side. My mom made this for me growing up because her aunt used to make it; I'll probably make it for my daughter and hope she likes it enough to keep the tradition going. Either way, you can add it to your repertoire now, too! Welcome to the family. **MAKES 4 SERVINGS**

PREP TIME: 10 minutes
COOK TIME: 1 hour

2 (10-ounce) packages fresh spinach

3 tablespoons butter

½ white onion, finely chopped

3 garlic cloves, minced

8 ounces ricotta cheese

1 cup shredded Monterey Jack cheese

¼ cup grated Parmesan cheese

Salt

Freshly ground black pepper

2 eggs, whisked

1. Preheat the oven to 350°F.

2. In a medium saucepan of boiling water, boil the spinach for 2 minutes. Drain and let cool before squeezing out as much excess liquid as possible. Chop it finely.

3. In a large skillet over medium heat, melt the butter.

4. Add the onion and garlic. Sauté for 5 to 7 minutes until the onion is softened and translucent.

5. Stir in the spinach. Cook for 1 minute then remove from the heat.

6. Stir in the ricotta, Monterey Jack, and Parmesan. Season with salt and pepper. Mix well to combine.

7. Add the eggs and stir to combine. Transfer the mixture to a pie dish and bake for 45 minutes or until set. Cool slightly and cut into slices or squares.

PER SERVING: Calories: 380;
Total carbs: 9g; **Net carbs: 6g, 8%;**
Total fat: 29g, 68%; Protein: 23g, 24%;
Fiber: 3g; Sugar: 2g

VARIATION 1: Calories: 383;
Total carbs: 10g; **Net carbs: 6g, 9%;**
Total fat: 30g, 69%; Protein: 22g, 22%;
Fiber: 4g; Sugar: 2g

VARIATION 2: Calories: 374;
Total carbs: 9g; **Net carbs: 7g, 9%;**
Total fat: 29g, 68%; Protein: 22g, 23%;
Fiber: 2g; Sugar: 3g

VARIATION 1 **ZIA'S SPINACH TORTA WITH FETA AND OLIVES:**
Use feta instead of Parmesan, and add ¼ cup sliced black olives
to the mixture.

VARIATION 2 **ZIA'S TORTA WITH SWISS CHARD:** If you're
looking to switch up your greens, use Swiss chard (or kale) instead
of spinach.

PERFECT PAIR: Serve a slice as a side to some Uncle Marty's Chicken
(page 90).

NO-CRUST SPINACH QUICHE

I am of the "just skip it" mind-set when it comes to keto and Paleo eating—by that I mean if there's an ingredient in a recipe that doesn't fit my macros or food values, I'll just skip it instead of trying to find a replacement. It can be easy to spend too much time and money on fancy ingredients that don't taste as good, so I'd rather just have the parts I like that work and forget the rest. Take this keto spinach quiche: what makes it keto? I just didn't make a crust!

MAKES 6 SERVINGS

PREP TIME: 10 minutes
COOK TIME: 35 minutes

4 tablespoons butter, divided

1 onion, diced

2 garlic cloves, minced

2 cups fresh spinach, chopped

Salt

Freshly ground black pepper

10 eggs

1 cup heavy (whipping) cream

2 cups shredded cheese (Colby-Monterey Jack is good), divided

PER SERVING: Calories: 483; Total carbs: 4g; **Net carbs: 4g, 3%; Total fat: 43g, 79%; Protein: 21g, 18%;** Fiber: 0g; Sugar: 1g

VARIATION 1: Calories: 682; Total carbs: 5g; **Net carbs: 5g, 2%; Total fat: 58g, 76%; Protein: 36g, 22%;** Fiber: 0g; Sugar: 1g

VARIATION 2: Calories: 496; Total carbs: 4g; **Net carbs: 4g, 3%; Total fat: 44g, 79%; Protein: 22g, 18%;** Fiber: 0g; Sugar: 1g

1. Preheat the oven to 375°F.

2. Grease a large round baking dish with 2 tablespoons of butter.

3. In a medium skillet over medium heat, combine the onion, garlic, spinach, and remaining 2 tablespoons of butter. Season with salt and pepper. Sauté for 4 to 5 minutes and remove from the heat.

4. In a large bowl, whisk the eggs and cream. Add the spinach and 1 cup of cheese and mix to combine. Pour the mixture into the prepared baking dish and season with more salt and pepper. Top with the remaining 1 cup of cheese. Bake for about 30 minutes or until the eggs are set. Cool slightly, slice, and serve. Refrigerate leftovers in an airtight container for up to 1 week.

VARIATION 1 **NO-CRUST BACON AND SPINACH QUICHE:** Add 8 ounces chopped cooked bacon to the quiche mixture before baking.

VARIATION 2 **NO-CRUST SPINACH QUICHE WITH FETA AND RED ONION:** Add a little more flavor to the quiche by topping the baked quiche with ¼ cup crumbled feta and ¼ red onion, thinly sliced.

KETO EGGS FLORENTINE (BENEDICT-STYLE)

The rich Hollandaise and runny yolk of the poached egg in this recipe is so luxurious that I don't even miss the English muffin it's usually served on. Eggs Florentine uses spinach instead of Canadian bacon, so it's a great vegetarian option for times you may not want meat. **MAKES 4 SERVINGS**

PREP TIME: 15 minutes
COOK TIME: 15 minutes

8 portobello mushroom caps

2 tablespoons extra-virgin olive oil

Salt

Freshly ground black pepper

Dash white vinegar

8 whole eggs

½ cup Creamed Spinach (page 204)

1 recipe Hollandaise Sauce (page 226)

PER SERVING: Calories: 593; Total carbs: 10g; **Net carbs: 6g, 6%; Total fat: 56g, 80%; Protein: 23g, 14%;** Fiber: 4g; Sugar: 1g

VARIATION 1: Calories: 599; Total carbs: 10g; **Net carbs: 7g, 5%; Total fat: 49g, 73%; Protein: 34g, 22%;** Fiber: 3g; Sugar: 1g

VARIATION 2: Calories: 579; Total carbs: 6g; **Net carbs: 4g, 4%; Total fat: 55g, 84%; Protein: 18g, 12%;** Fiber:2 g; Sugar: 4g

1. Place a grill pan or large skillet over medium heat. Brush both sides of each portobello mushroom with olive oil and season with salt and pepper. Cook for 3 minutes per side. Remove from the heat and set aside.

2. Bring a large saucepan of water to a low simmer. Add the vinegar. Crack 1 egg into a small dish. Use a large spoon to swirl the simmering water into a slow whirlpool. Carefully drop the egg into the water and, without hitting the egg, continue the swirling motion with the spoon. Cook for 1 to 2 minutes until the white sets. Carefully scoop the egg out and place it on a paper towel. Repeat with the remaining eggs.

3. To assemble the eggs Benedict, place the mushroom caps on plates, bottom-side facing up. Add the creamed spinach and top with a poached egg and some Hollandaise.

VARIATION 1 **REGULAR (KETO/PALEO) EGGS BENEDICT:** Instead of spinach, add 1 slice grilled Canadian bacon to each mushroom cap before topping with an egg and some Hollandaise.

VARIATION 2 **EGGS BENEDICT ON TOMATO SLICES:** If you don't have the time or desire to grill portobello mushrooms, serve these Benedicts on sliced tomatoes.

LOW-CARB GREEN SMOOTHIE

Smoothies make a great breakfast or mid-morning snack. But when you're keto, your options are limited because fruit is high in carbs. This version is mostly almond milk and spinach, with a few fresh raspberries for sweetness and fruitiness. The cream cheese adds a luscious richness and makes this smoothie taste almost like a milk shake! **MAKES 1 SMOOTHIE**

PREP TIME: 5 minutes
COOK TIME: 0 minutes

1 cup almond milk

1½ cups fresh spinach

¼ cup fresh raspberries

1 ounce cream cheese

Ice

PER SERVING: Calories: 156;
Total carbs: 8g; **Net carbs: 4g, 17%;**
Total fat: 13g, 73%; Protein: 4g, 9%;
Fiber: 4g; Sugar: 2g

VARIATION 1: Calories: 177;
Total carbs: 7g; **Net carbs: 3g, 13%;**
Total fat: 17g, 83%; Protein: 2g, 4%;
Fiber: 4g; Sugar: 2g

VARIATION 2: Calories: 180;
Total carbs: 14g; **Net carbs: 7g, 19%;**
Total fat: 14g, 71%; Protein: 6g, 10%;
Fiber: 7g; Sugar: 2g

In a blender, combine the almond milk, spinach, raspberries, cream cheese, and a handful of ice. Blend until smooth and serve immediately.

VARIATION 1 **DAIRY-FREE LOW-CARB GREEN SMOOTHIE:** Skip the cream cheese and add 1 tablespoon coconut oil.

VARIATION 2 **LOW-CARB RASPBERRY CHOCOLATE SMOOTHIE:** Add 2 tablespoons unsweetened cocoa powder or your favorite keto-friendly chocolate protein powder.

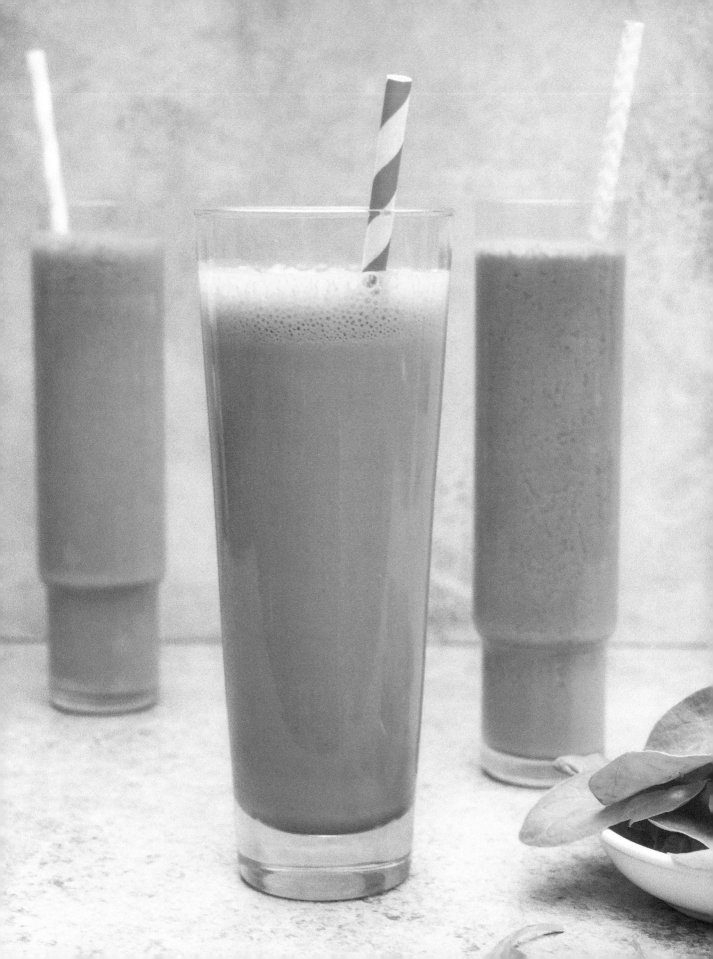

KETO SPINACH ARTICHOKE DIP

This is the easiest way to make spinach artichoke dip, which is one of my all-time favorite snacks and appetizers. If you have a party and serve this, you know where to find me—stuffing my face with it. It's great on its own, on top of chicken, or with sliced veggies for dipping instead of the more traditional high-carb toast or crackers. **MAKES 6 SERVINGS**

PREP TIME: 5 minutes
COOK TIME: 10 minutes

1 cup frozen chopped spinach, thawed and drained

1½ cups canned artichoke hearts, drained and chopped

Salt

Freshly ground black pepper

8 ounces cream cheese

¼ cup sour cream

¼ cup Keto Mayonnaise (page 225)

⅓ cup grated Parmesan cheese

1 teaspoon garlic powder

1 teaspoon red pepper flakes

PER SERVING: Calories: 223;
Total carbs: 7g; **Net carbs: 6g, 10%;**
Total fat: 20g, 80%; Protein: 6g, 10%;
Fiber: 1g; Sugar: 2g

VARIATION 1: Calories: 223;
Total carbs: 7g; **Net carbs: 6g, 10%;**
Total fat: 20g, 80%; Protein: 6g, 10%;
Fiber: 1g; Sugar: 2g

VARIATION 2: Calories: 223;
Total carbs: 7g; **Net carbs: 6g, 10%;**
Total fat: 20g, 80%; Protein: 6g, 10%;
Fiber: 1g; Sugar: 2g

1. In a small saucepan over medium-low heat, combine the spinach and artichokes. Season with salt and pepper.

2. Add the cream cheese and stir to combine until completely melted. Remove from the heat and stir in the sour cream, mayonnaise, Parmesan, garlic powder, and red pepper flakes. Serve hot.

VARIATION 1 **BAKED SPINACH ARTICHOKE DIP:** Mix together all the ingredients in an 8- or 9-inch square baking dish and top with ¼ cup shredded mozzarella. Bake at 350°F for 20 minutes or until the cheese melts.

VARIATION 2 **SLOW COOKER SPINACH AND ARTICHOKE DIP:** If you want to make a double batch ahead of time, mix everything together and cook in your slow cooker on low heat for 2 hours.

MAKE AHEAD: Make this dip a few days ahead of time and store in a covered baking dish. Before serving, top it with more Parmesan and bake at 350°F for 15 to 20 minutes.

CHEESY SPINACH PUFFS

These little cheesy spinach balls are a great keto appetizer to bring to your next potluck, which is something I like to do to make sure there's at least one thing I can eat (although there's usually a charcuterie or cheese board around somewhere, which is all I really need). They also make a great snack, so prepare a double batch and keep them in the refrigerator for those times between meals when you could really go for something tasty. **MAKES ABOUT 8 SERVINGS**

PREP TIME: 10 minutes
COOK TIME: 10 minutes
CHILLING TIME: 10 minutes

`30` `GF`

16 ounces frozen spinach, thawed, drained, and squeezed of as much excess liquid as possible

1 cup almond flour

4 tablespoons butter, melted, plus more for the baking sheet

2 eggs

¼ cup grated Parmesan cheese

¼ cup cream cheese

3 tablespoons heavy (whipping) cream

1 tablespoon onion powder

1 teaspoon garlic powder

Salt

Freshly ground black pepper

PER SERVING: Calories: 159;
Total carbs: 3g; **Net carbs: 1g, 8%;**
Total fat: 14g, 78%; Protein: 6g, 14%;
Fiber: 2g; Sugar: 1g

VARIATION 1: Calories: 147;
Total carbs: 3g; **Net carbs: 1g, 9%;**
Total fat: 13g, 76%; Protein: 6g, 15%;
Fiber: 2g; Sugar: 1g

VARIATION 2: Calories: 200;
Total carbs: 3g; **Net carbs: 1g, 7%;**
Total fat: 17g, 76%; Protein: 9g, 17%;
Fiber: 2g; Sugar: 1g

1. In a food processor, combine the spinach, almond flour, butter, eggs, Parmesan, cream cheese, cream, onion powder, and garlic powder. Season with salt and pepper. Blend until smooth. Transfer to the refrigerator and chill for 10 to 15 minutes.

2. Preheat the oven to 350°F.

3. Grease a baking sheet with butter.

4. Scoop the spinach mixture in heaping tablespoons and roll into balls. Place on the prepared baking sheet and bake for about 10 minutes until set. When tapped with your finger, they should not still be soft. Enjoy warm (best!) or cold. Refrigerate in an air-tight container for up to 4 days.

`VARIATION 1` **CHEESY FETA SPINACH PUFFS:** Use feta instead of cream cheese.

`VARIATION 2` **CHEESY BACON SPINACH PUFFS:** Top these puffs with crumbled cooked bacon.

CREAMED SPINACH

This is a really easy way to make spinach super delicious. (Spoiler alert— anytime I say that, it usually involves cream cheese.) I don't often have creamed spinach unless I'm out at a barbecue place, but this recipe is so simple it's hard to resist. I like it as a side dish with any dinner entrée, but it's even good with some scrambled eggs in the morning! **MAKES 4 SERVINGS**

PREP TIME: 5 minutes
COOK TIME: 20 minutes

10 ounces fresh spinach

2 tablespoons butter

½ onion, minced

3 garlic cloves, minced

Salt

Freshly ground black pepper

4 ounces cream cheese, cubed

½ cup heavy (whipping) cream

PER SERVING: Calories: 272; Total carbs: 6g; **Net carbs: 4g, 8%; Total fat: 27g, 86%; Protein: 5g, 6%;** Fiber: 2g; Sugar: 2g

VARIATION 1: Calories: 464; Total carbs: 6g; **Net carbs: 4g, 5%; Total fat: 46g, 87%; Protein: 9g, 8%;** Fiber: 2g; Sugar: 2g

VARIATION 2: Calories: 382; Total carbs: 17g; **Net carbs: 11g, 16%; Total fat: 34g, 78%; Protein: 7g, 6%;** Fiber: 6g; Sugar: 3g

1. In a large saucepan of boiling water, cook the spinach for 1 to 2 minutes or until wilted. Remove from the water, drain, cool, and squeeze out as much excess liquid as possible.

2. In the same pan over medium heat, melt the butter.

3. Add the onion and garlic. Season with salt and pepper. Sauté for 5 to 7 minutes until the onion is softened and translucent.

4. Add the cream cheese a little at a time and let it melt.

5. Stir in the cream to combine. Reduce the heat to medium low. Bring the mixture to a low simmer and add the spinach. Cook for 8 to 10 minutes or until hot and thick. Season again with salt and pepper and serve hot. Refrigerate leftovers in an airtight container for up to 3 days.

VARIATION 1 **CREAMED SPINACH WITH PANCETTA:** Sauté the onion and garlic together with 6 to 8 ounces diced pancetta instead of the butter. Follow the rest of the recipe as written.

VARIATION 2 **CREAMED KALE WITH AVOCADO:** Use kale instead of spinach and top with sliced avocado.

SAUTÉED SPINACH WITH GARLIC

My mom went to a yoga retreat at a place called Yogaville several years ago when I was in college, and I visited her there for dinner one night—the food was all vegetarian and not really my thing, but for some reason I still remember the spinach they served. It was really garlicky and delicious and I just couldn't stop thinking about it, so I finally made my own. **MAKES 4 SERVINGS**

PREP TIME: 5 minutes
COOK TIME: 10 minutes

2 tablespoons butter, or olive oil

¼ white onion, diced

3 garlic cloves, sliced

12 ounces fresh spinach

Salt

Freshly ground black pepper

PER SERVING: Calories: 75;
Total carbs: 4g; **Net carbs: 2g, 20%;**
Total fat: 6g, 71%; Protein: 3g, 9%;
Fiber: 2g; Sugar: 1g

VARIATION 1: Calories: 102;
Total carbs: 5g; **Net carbs: 3g, 16%;**
Total fat: 8g, 67%; Protein: 5g, 17%;
Fiber: 2g; Sugar: 1g

VARIATION 2: Calories: 171;
Total carbs: 4g; **Net carbs: 2g, 9%;**
Total fat: 16g, 81%; Protein: 5g, 10%;
Fiber: 2g; Sugar: 1g

1. In a large skillet over medium heat, melt the butter.

2. Add the onion and garlic. Cook for 5 to 7 minutes until the onion is softened and translucent.

3. Add the spinach and reduce the heat to medium low. Season well with salt and pepper. Cook for 3 to 4 minutes or until the spinach wilts. Serve immediately.

VARIATION 1 **SAUTÉED SPINACH WITH GARLIC AND CHEESE:** Add ¼ cup grated Parmesan to the spinach before serving. Stir well to combine.

VARIATION 2 **SAUTÉED SPINACH WITH GARLIC AND BACON:** Cook 2 or 3 bacon slices in the skillet before adding the garlic and onion. Remove the bacon and crumble it. Add the spinach and return the bacon to the skillet. Stir well to combine.

PERFECT PAIR: Serve with Keto Sloppy Joes (page 103).

WARM SPINACH SALAD

This is an easy go-to salad that doesn't have too many ingredients, so it's perfect if you're home for lunch or want to make a quick salad to go with your dinner. It's also easy to customize, so feel free to switch up the dressings or add some cheese if you've got it. **MAKES 2 SERVINGS**

PREP TIME: 10 minutes
COOK TIME: 5 minutes

2 cups fresh spinach leaves

½ cucumber, quartered and sliced

2 or 3 bacon slices, cut widthwise into strips

¼ red onion, thinly sliced

3 to 4 tablespoons Ranch Dressing (page 225)

PER SERVING: Calories: 229;
Total carbs: 7g; **Net carbs: 6g, 11%;**
Total fat: 20g, 79%; Protein: 6g, 10%;
Fiber: 1g; Sugar: 3g

VARIATION 1: Calories: 229;
Total carbs: 7g; **Net carbs: 6g, 11%;**
Total fat: 20g, 79%; Protein: 6g, 10%;
Fiber: 1g; Sugar: 3g

VARIATION 2: Calories: 411;
Total carbs: 19g; **Net carbs: 9g, 16%;**
Total fat: 36g, 75%; Protein: 10g, 9%;
Fiber: 10g; Sugar: 6g

1. In a large bowl, combine the spinach and cucumber.

2. In a medium skillet over medium-high heat, sauté the bacon and onion together for 4 to 5 minutes until the bacon is crisp and the onion is caramelized. With a slotted spoon, remove the bacon and onion and add to the spinach and cucumber.

3. Pour the dressing over the salad and toss to coat.

VARIATION 1 **SPINACH SALAD:** Skip the stove and use cooked bacon from the refrigerator.

VARIATION 2 **SPINACH SALAD WITH AVOCADO:** Make either the warm or cold salad (Variation 1) and top with 1 large avocado, diced, for some extra fat.

CHICKEN FLORENTINE

I love this Chicken Florentine recipe—it's creamy and delicious, but loaded with spinach, so you can feel good about getting some protein, lots of fat, and a nice serving of greens all at the same time. It also can be partially made ahead of time and then baked in the oven until you're ready to serve, which makes it a perfect family dinner for a busy weeknight. **MAKES 4 SERVINGS**

PREP TIME: 10 minutes
COOK TIME: 30 minutes

1 pound boneless skinless chicken breasts

Salt

Freshly ground black pepper

3 tablespoons butter, divided

¼ white onion, diced

2 garlic cloves, minced

1 cup chicken broth

1 cup heavy (whipping) cream

10 ounces fresh spinach, chopped

½ cup grated Parmesan cheese

PER SERVING: Calories: 489; Total carbs: 6g; **Net carbs: 4g, 5%;** **Total fat: 36g, 65%; Protein: 36g, 30%;** Fiber: 2g; Sugar: 1g

VARIATION 1: Calories: 495; Total carbs: 8g; **Net carbs: 6g, 6%;** **Total fat: 36g, 64%; Protein: 36g, 30%;** Fiber: 2g; Sugar: 2g

VARIATION 2: Calories: 380; Total carbs: 9g; **Net carbs: 7g, 8%;** **Total fat: 35g, 81%; Protein: 12g, 11%;** Fiber: 2g; Sugar: 2g

1. Preheat the oven to 200°F.

2. Season the chicken with salt and pepper. In a large skillet over medium heat, melt 1½ tablespoons of butter. Add the chicken and cook for about 5 minutes per side or until browned. Transfer the chicken to an ovenproof dish and keep it warm in the low oven.

3. Return the skillet to the heat and melt the remaining 1½ tablespoons of butter.

4. Add the onion and garlic. Sauté for 5 to 7 minutes until the onion is softened and translucent.

5. Add the chicken broth. Increase the heat to medium high and simmer for about 3 minutes until reduced slightly

6. Stir in the cream and spinach. Cook for 3 to 4 minutes. Transfer the sauce to the baking dish with the chicken. Top with the Parmesan. Increase the oven temperature to 350°F. Cook for about 5 minutes or until the Parmesan browns slightly. Refrigerate leftovers in an airtight container for up to 5 days.

VARIATION 1 **CHICKEN FLORENTINE WITH VEGGIES:** Add some more veggies to your plate by sautéing ½ red bell pepper, diced, and 1 carrot, diced, with the garlic and onion.

VARIATION 2 **MUSHROOMS FLORENTINE:** Make this a vegetarian dish by using 1 pound sliced mushrooms instead of chicken.

ALLERGEN TIP: Skip the Parmesan and use coconut cream instead of heavy cream to make this a dairy-free version.

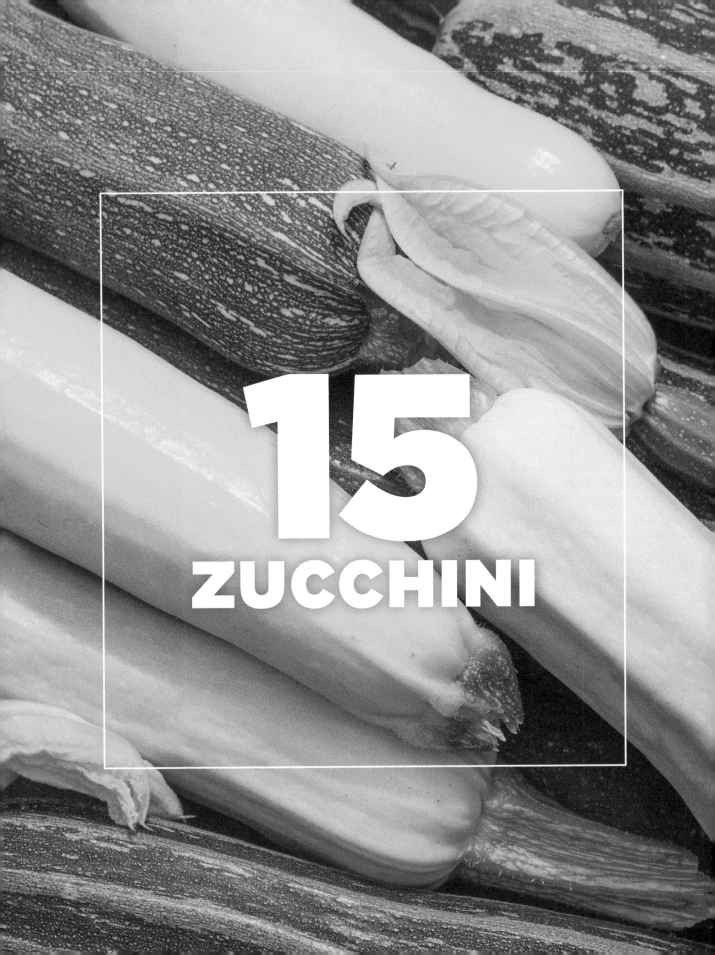

15
ZUCCHINI

Zucchini is kind of an all-star when it comes to Paleo and keto cooking—it's full of nutrients, low in carbs, and a versatile ingredient (not to mention one of the easiest to turn into noodles when you're really craving some pasta). Other than spinach, zucchini is the only other vegetable I always buy at the store no matter what; I know that even without planning, I'm going to end up using it in some way every week.

From the simplest use, tossed into some bone broth as a quick noodle soup, to the most labor-intensive Zucchini Lasagna (page 212), zucchini is a delicious way to add texture, flavor, and vitamins to your keto meals.

ZUCCHINI NOODLE SALAD

This zucchini noodle, or "zoodle," salad is a really fun take on classic salads with spinach or lettuce leaves. I had forgotten how good zucchini can be when eaten raw, and I especially enjoy it in noodle form. Add a few more veggies and some dressing and you've got a really colorful, interesting salad!

MAKES 2 SERVINGS

PREP TIME: 15 minutes
COOK TIME: 0 minutes

2 large zucchini, spiralized or peeled into thin strips

1 small tomato, diced

¼ red onion, sliced thinly

1 large avocado, diced

½ cup olive oil

¼ cup balsamic vinegar

1 garlic clove, minced

2 teaspoons Dijon mustard

Salt

Freshly ground black pepper

¼ cup blue cheese crumbles

1. In a large bowl, combine the zucchini noodles, tomato, onion, and avocado.

2. In a small bowl, whisk together the olive oil, vinegar, garlic, mustard, and some salt and pepper. Drizzle over the salad and toss to combine. Divide into serving bowls and top with the blue cheese crumbles.

VARIATION 1 **ZUCCHINI NOODLE SALAD WITH GRILLED CHICKEN:** Serve this salad with ½ pound chopped grilled chicken breasts or thighs.

VARIATION 2 **SUMMER SQUASH NOODLE SALAD:** Swap yellow squash for the zucchini.

ALLERGEN TIP: Omit the blue cheese crumbles if you don't tolerate dairy.

PER SERVING: Calories: 770; Total carbs: 22g; **Net carbs: 12g, 11%;** **Total fat: 75g, 85%; Protein: 8g, 4%;** Fiber: 10g; Sugar: 11g

VARIATION 1: Calories: 956; Total carbs: 22g; **Net carbs: 12g, 9%;** **Total fat: 79g, 72%; Protein: 43g, 19%;** Fiber: 10g; Sugar: 11g

VARIATION 2: Calories: 770; Total carbs: 22g; **Net carbs: 12g, 11%;** **Total fat: 75g, 85%; Protein: 8g, 4%;** Fiber: 10g; Sugar: 11g

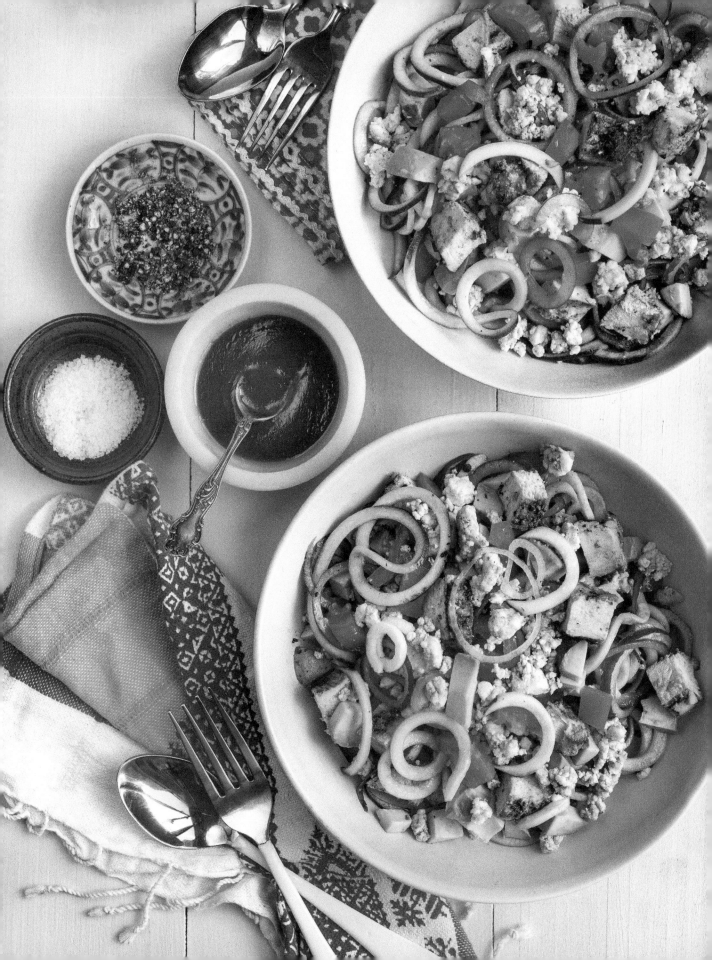

ZUCCHINI LASAGNA

This lasagna started out as a Paleo recipe my mom and I created, but now that I eat more keto I'm able to add some cheese to it, which really brings it together beautifully. It's a little time-intensive but you can make a lot of it ahead of time and then just pop it in the oven on a Sunday evening so you can relax. **MAKES 6 SERVINGS**

PREP TIME: 15 minutes
COOK TIME: 1 hour, 20 minutes

1 pound spicy Italian sausage, casings removed

1 pound ground beef

Salt

Freshly ground black pepper

1 small green bell pepper, diced

1 onion, diced

1 (16-ounce) can no-sugar-added tomato sauce

2 tablespoons tomato paste

2 tablespoons chopped fresh parsley leaves

2 tablespoons chopped fresh basil leaves

1 tablespoon chopped fresh oregano leaves

2 large zucchini, cut lengthwise with a peeler into thin sheets that resemble lasagna noodles

8 ounces ricotta cheese

½ cup shredded mozzarella cheese, plus more for topping

1. Preheat the oven to 325°F.

2. In a large skillet over medium heat, cook the sausage for 5 to 7 minutes, crumbling with a wooden spoon, until done. Transfer to a plate and set aside.

3. Return the skillet to medium heat and add the beef. Cook for 5 minutes, using a wooden spoon to break up the meat. Season with salt and pepper.

4. Add the bell pepper and onion. Continue to cook for 5 to 7 minutes until the beef is no longer pink.

5. Stir in the tomato sauce, tomato paste, parsley, basil, and oregano. Season with salt and pepper. Once the sauce begins to boil, reduce the heat to low and simmer for 20 minutes, stirring frequently. Remove from the heat.

6. To assemble the lasagna: Spread half the meat sauce into the bottom of a 9-by-13-inch baking dish. Layer half the zucchini slices over the meat sauce. Add half the sausage. Spread half the ricotta on top and sprinkle with half the mozzarella. Make another layer in the same order. Cover with aluminum foil and bake for 45 minutes.

7. Remove the foil and increase the oven temperature to 375°F. Top with more mozzarella and bake for 10 to 15 minutes more. Remove from the oven and let rest for 5 minutes before slicing. Serve warm. Cover and refrigerate leftovers for up to 4 days.

PER SERVING: Calories: 483;
Total carbs: 6g; **Net carbs: 5g, 5%;**
Total fat: 37g, 67%; Protein: 33g, 28%;
Fiber: 1g; Sugar: 3g

VARIATION 1: Calories: 503;
Total carbs: 9g; **Net carbs: 7g, 6%;**
Total fat: 37g, 66%; Protein: 36g, 28%;
Fiber: 2g; Sugar: 4g

VARIATION 2: Calories: 150;
Total carbs: 13g; **Net carbs: 8g, 31%;**
Total fat: 8g, 44%; Protein: 10g, 35%;
Fiber: 5g; Sugar: 6g

VARIATION 1 **ZUCCHINI LASAGNA WITH MUSHROOMS:** Add 1 pound sliced fresh mushrooms to the meat sauce.

VARIATION 2 **VEGETARIAN ZUCCHINI LASAGNA:** Skip the meat sauce and sausage filling and use mushrooms and eggplant instead (about 1 pound each). Dice the eggplant and cook it as in step 2, instead of the sausage. Incorporate the mushrooms into the sauce in step 4. Follow the rest of the recipe as written.

EASY PEANUT ZOODLES

This is my go-to recipe when I crave Thai food but don't want to mess up my whole day with a cheat meal. The only part that actually takes time is salting the zoodles, which helps them stay crunchy through the cooking process. If you do that ahead of time you've got a recipe that only takes 10 minutes— perfect for dinner on a busy day or a quick lunch at home between work or errands. **MAKES 2 SERVINGS**

PREP TIME: 10 minutes
COOK TIME: 5 minutes
DRAINING TIME: 15 minutes

2 large zucchini, spiralized or peeled into thin strips

Salt

1 teaspoon sesame oil

1 garlic clove, minced

1 teaspoon red pepper flakes

1 tablespoon gluten-free soy sauce

3 tablespoons unsweetened peanut butter

2 to 3 tablespoons chicken broth (optional)

Freshly ground black pepper

2 tablespoons crushed peanuts

2 tablespoons chopped fresh cilantro leaves

2 lime wedges

PER SERVING: Calories: 221; Total carbs: 8g; **Net carbs: 6g, 11%;** **Total fat: 18g, 72%; Protein: 10g, 17%;** Fiber: 2g; Sugar: 2g

VARIATION 1: Calories: 308; Total carbs: 8g; **Net carbs: 6g, 8%;** **Total fat: 19g, 54%; Protein: 28g, 34%;** Fiber: 2g; Sugar: 2g

VARIATION 2: Calories: 313; Total carbs: 8g; **Net carbs: 6g, 8%;** **Total fat: 19g, 53%; Protein: 29g, 39%;** Fiber: 2g; Sugar: 2g

1. Place the zucchini noodles in a colander and sprinkle liberally with salt. Let sit in the sink for 15 to 20 minutes before rinsing and patting dry with a paper towel.

2. While the zucchini is draining, in a large skillet over medium-low heat, heat the sesame oil.

3. Add the garlic and red pepper flakes. Cook for 2 to 3 minutes until fragrant.

4. Stir in the soy sauce and peanut butter.

5. Add the zucchini noodles and toss to combine, ensuring that sauce coats all of the noodles. (If the sauce is too thick, add some chicken broth to thin it.) Season with salt and pepper and transfer to two bowls to serve.

6. Top with the crushed peanuts and cilantro and serve with the lime wedges.

VARIATION 1 EASY PEANUT ZOODLES WITH SHRIMP: Add ½ cup cooked shrimp to the pan and toss to combine until warmed through.

VARIATION 2 EASY PEANUT ZOODLES WITH CHICKEN: Add 1 large boneless skinless chicken breast, sliced, to the pan to cook with the garlic and red pepper flakes. Cook for 5 to 7 minutes or until browned and cooked through. Follow the rest of the recipe as written. (You can also use steamed chicken or a rotisserie chicken if you have it handy.)

MAKE IT PALEO: Use almond butter and coconut aminos instead of peanut butter and soy sauce.

TACO ZUCCHINI BOATS

These boats are a fun way to incorporate zucchini into a meal that otherwise might not have enough vegetables (and to get kids to eat their veggies!). I use similar ingredients when I'm making taco salads, but in this recipe I transfer the meat and cheese into hollowed-out zucchini boats, which are topped with more cheese and baked until nice and hot and flavorful. **MAKES 4 SERVINGS**

PREP TIME: 10 minutes
COOK TIME: 1 hour

1 pound ground beef

4 large zucchini, halved lengthwise

2 tablespoons olive oil

1 onion, diced

2 garlic cloves, minced

Salt

Freshly ground black pepper

1½ teaspoons chili powder

1 teaspoon ground cumin

¼ cup salsa

1 cup shredded Mexican blend cheese, divided

1 avocado, diced

2 to 3 tablespoons chopped fresh cilantro leaves

¼ cup sour cream

PER SERVING: Calories: 499; Total carbs: 11g; **Net carbs: 6g, 8%; Total fat: 38g, 67%; Protein: 31g, 25%;** Fiber: 5g; Sugar: 4g

VARIATION 1: Calories: 550; Total carbs: 11g; **Net carbs: 6g, 7%; Total fat: 43g, 68%; Protein: 34g, 25%;** Fiber: 5g; Sugar: 4g

VARIATION 2: Calories: 504; Total carbs: 11g; **Net carbs: 6g, 8%; Total fat: 38g, 67%; Protein: 31g, 25%;** Fiber: 5g; Sugar: 4g

1. Preheat the oven to 350°F.

2. Put the beef in a large bowl.

3. With a spoon, scoop out the zucchini flesh, chop it, and add it to the beef. Set the zucchini shells (boats) aside.

4. In a skillet over medium-high heat, heat the olive oil.

5. Add the onion and garlic. Sauté for 5 to 7 minutes until the onion is softened and translucent.

6. Add the beef and zucchini mixture and cook for 5 to 7 minutes until the beef is completely browned, breaking the meat up as you cook it. Season with salt, pepper, chili powder, and cumin. Remove the skillet from the heat.

7. Stir in the salsa and ½ cup of cheese. Stir well.

8. Stuff the zucchini boats with the meat mixture. Top with the remaining ½ cup of cheese. Place them on a baking sheet and bake for 45 minutes.

9. Remove from the oven and top each with avocado slices, cilantro, and a dollop of sour cream.

VARIATION 1 **GRANDMA'S ZUCCHINI BOATS:** Instead of taco seasonings, add ¾ cup sliced green olives and 2 chopped hardboiled eggs to the meat mixture.

VARIATION 2 **SPICY TACO ZUCCHINI BOATS:** Add ½ diced jalapeño pepper to the skillet with the onion and garlic, and use pepper jack instead of the cheese blend.

MAKE AHEAD: Cook everything, stuff the zucchini, and refrigerate until ready to bake.

ZUCCHINI PIZZA BITES

These fabulous little zucchini pizza bites are a little quicker to make than Cauliflower Pizza (page 166), and just as good. Plus, they have a snack-y quality that's just great when you're having friends over but maybe didn't plan to make a full meal. For this recipe, it's best to get the largest zucchini you can find so you have plenty of surface area to make your mini pizzas.

MAKES 4 SERVINGS

PREP TIME: 10 minutes
COOK TIME: 15 minutes

3 or 4 large zucchini, cut into ½-inch-thick rounds

Salt

Freshly ground black pepper

½ cup no-sugar-added pizza sauce

1 cup shredded mozzarella cheese

12 ounces sliced pepperoni

PER SERVING: Calories: 505; Total carbs: 2g; **Net carbs: 2g, 1%;** **Total fat: 43g, 77%; Protein: 26g, 22%;** Fiber: 0g; Sugar: 1g

VARIATION 1: Calories: 536; Total carbs: 9g; **Net carbs: 4g, 6%;** **Total fat: 44g, 73%; Protein: 27g, 21%;** Fiber: 5g; Sugar: 4g

VARIATION 2: Calories: 147; Total carbs: 6g; **Net carbs: 4g, 15%;** **Total fat: 11g, 65%; Protein: 7g, 20%;** Fiber: 2g; Sugar: 1g

1. Preheat the oven to 350°F.

2. Arrange the zucchini rounds on a baking sheet. Season with salt and pepper.

3. Spoon pizza sauce onto each round and add a pinch or two of mozzarella.

4. Top with pepperoni (you may have to chop it if space is limited). Bake for 15 to 20 minutes or until the cheese melts.

VARIATION 1 **MINI EGGPLANT PIZZAS:** Use sliced eggplant instead of zucchini.

VARIATION 2 **VEGETARIAN PIZZA BITES:** Skip the pepperoni and use sliced black olives instead.

ZUCCHINI FRIES WITH GARLIC AIOLI

This recipe is such a great way to enjoy zucchini. I love how crispy they get with the seasoned almond flour, and I can't seem to get enough of the garlic aioli dipping sauce (which is probably why I suggest you serve it not only with these fries, but also with my Keto Fish Cakes on page 126...and really anything else your heart desires). They make a great appetizer or a side dish, so make sure to try them soon, whether you're preparing a big dinner for friends or just in the mood for a healthy snack. **MAKES 4 SERVINGS**

PREP TIME: 10 minutes
COOK TIME: 20 minutes

2 eggs, whisked

½ cup almond flour

1½ teaspoons onion powder

1½ teaspoons garlic powder

1 teaspoon red pepper flakes

2 large zucchini, ends trimmed, halved widthwise then lengthwise, and cut into French fry–like strips

Salt

Freshly ground black pepper

½ cup garlic aioli (see Keto Fish Cakes with Garlic Aioli, page 126)

PER SERVING: Calories: 173; Total carbs: 8g; **Net carbs: 7g, 18%;** **Total fat: 14g, 70%; Protein: 4g, 12%;** Fiber: 1g; Sugar: 2g

VARIATION 1: Calories: 263; Total carbs: 8g; **Net carbs: 7g, 12%;** **Total fat: 24g, 80%; Protein: 4g, 8%;** Fiber: 1g; Sugar: 2g

VARIATION 2: Calories: 193; Total carbs: 11g; **Net carbs: 9g, 23%;** **Total fat: 14g, 65%; Protein: 6g, 12%;** Fiber: 3g; Sugar: 3g

1. Preheat the oven to 400°F.

2. Pour the eggs into a shallow bowl.

3. In a second shallow bowl, stir together the almond flour, onion powder, garlic powder, and red pepper flakes.

4. Pat the zucchini strips dry with a paper towel. Dip the zucchini fries first into the egg and then toss them in the seasoned almond flour. Season with salt and pepper and place on a rimmed baking sheet. Put the fries in the oven and immediately lower the heat to 350°F. Cook for about 20 minutes or until crisp. Check on the fries halfway through the cooking time and lower the heat if they're browning too quickly.

5. Serve with the garlic aioli.

VARIATION 1 **PANFRIED ZUCCHINI FRIES WITH GARLIC AIOLI:** Instead of baking in the oven, fry the zucchini in batches in a large skillet with 2 to 3 tablespoons of olive oil over medium-high heat for 2 to 3 minutes per side.

VARIATION 2 **BROCCOLI FRIES WITH GARLIC AIOLI:** Use broccoli florets instead of zucchini.

OLD-SCHOOL BUTTERED (ZUCCHINI) NOODLES

Sometimes simple is best—and these old-school buttered zoodles are no exception. Inspired by the pasta with butter and Parmesan I used to have as a kid, this is a veggie-packed version I can make anytime I feel the need for some comfort food. And because I always buy zucchini at the store and pretty much always have butter and Parmesan in my refrigerator, I can whip this dish up anytime as an easy lunch or snack. **MAKES 2 SERVINGS**

PREP TIME: 20 minutes
COOK TIME: 10 minutes
DRAINING TIME: 15 minutes

2 medium zucchini, spiralized or peeled into thin strips

Salt

3 tablespoons butter

1 garlic clove, minced

¼ cup grated Parmesan cheese

Freshly ground black pepper

Fresh parsley leaves, chopped, for garnish

PER SERVING: Calories: 209; Total carbs: 2g; **Net carbs: 2g, 2%;** **Total fat: 21g, 87%; Protein: 5g, 11%;** Fiber: 0g; Sugar: 0g

VARIATION 1: Calories: 240; Total carbs: 2g; **Net carbs: 2g, 3%;** **Total fat: 24g, 88%; Protein: 5g, 9%;** Fiber: 0g; Sugar: 0g

VARIATION 2: Calories: 523; Total carbs: 17g; **Net carbs: 13g, 11%;** **Total fat: 39g, 66%; Protein: 31g, 23%;** Fiber: 4g; Sugar: 10g

1. Place the zucchini noodles in a colander and sprinkle liberally with salt. Let them sit in the sink for 15 to 20 minutes before rinsing and patting dry with a paper towel.

2. In a large skillet over medium-low heat, melt the butter.

3. Add the garlic and sauté for 3 to 4 minutes.

4. Add the zucchini noodles, toss to combine, and cook for 5 to 6 minutes or until softened. Season with salt and pepper. Remove from the heat and top with the Parmesan and some freshly chopped parsley.

VARIATION 1 **AGLIO E OLIO:** Use olive oil instead of butter and add an extra garlic clove. Sauté the garlic in the oil and add 1 teaspoon red pepper flakes. Add the zucchini noodles and cook for 4 to 5 minutes over medium heat. Top with Parmesan, parsley, and a squeeze of fresh lemon juice.

VARIATION 2 **EASY ZOODLES WITH MEAT SAUCE:** Skip the butter and use only olive oil. Sauté ½ pound ground beef with a small (6-ounce) can of tomato paste and the garlic over medium heat for 5 to 6 minutes or until browned. Add the zucchini noodles and cook for 5 minutes more. Top with Parmesan, parsley, and serve.

CHEESY ZUCCHINI GRATIN

This cheesy zucchini gratin is an incredibly luxurious side dish that you and your family are sure to love. What could be bad about veggies topped with a decadent cheese sauce? **MAKES 6 SERVINGS**

PREP TIME: 10 minutes
COOK TIME: 40 minutes

4 tablespoons butter

1 large onion, sliced

2 garlic cloves, minced

1 cup heavy (whipping) cream

¼ cup cream cheese

Salt

Freshly ground black pepper

4 or 5 large zucchini, cut into ¼-inch-thick rounds

¾ cup shredded white Cheddar cheese

PER SERVING: Calories: 307; Total carbs: 5g; **Net carbs: 4g, 6%;** **Total fat: 30g, 87%; Protein: 6g, 7%;** Fiber: 1g; Sugar: 2g

VARIATION 1: Calories: 306; Total carbs: 5g; **Net carbs: 4g, 6%;** **Total fat: 30g, 86%; Protein: 6g, 8%;** Fiber: 1g; Sugar: 2g

VARIATION 2: Calories: 494; Total carbs: 5g; **Net carbs: 4g, 4%;** **Total fat: 34g, 61%; Protein: 41g, 35%;** Fiber:1 g; Sugar: 2g

1. In a large saucepan over medium-low heat, melt the butter.

2. Add the onion and garlic. Cook for about 15 minutes until the garlic is fragrant and the onion begins to caramelize. Reduce the heat to low.

3. Stir in the cream. Simmer for 2 minutes.

4. Add the cream cheese. Season with salt and pepper. Stir until smooth.

5. Place the zucchini in a 7-by-11-inch baking dish and cover with the cream sauce. Top with the Cheddar and bake for about 20 minutes or until the cheese melts and turns golden brown. Cool slightly before serving. Refrigerate leftovers in an airtight container for up to 4 days.

VARIATION 1 **CHEESY ZUCCHINI GRATIN WITH GRUYÈRE:** Give this gratin a fancier spin with Gruyère instead of Cheddar.

VARIATION 2 **ZUCCHINI GRATIN WITH CHICKEN:** Make this a one-pot meal by adding 1½ pounds diced cooked boneless skinless chicken breasts to the baking dish with the zucchini. Cover with the sauce and follow the rest of the recipe as written.

PERFECT PAIR: Serve as a side with Steak and Mushroom Kebabs (page 97).

LOW-CARB ZUCCHINI FRITTERS

These zucchini fritters are my take on keto hash browns—they get crispy and are great to have in the refrigerator to reheat with virtually anything: eggs, chicken, salads, or even just as a snack with some Garlic Aioli (see Keto Fish Cakes with Garlic Aioli, page 126). **MAKES 4 SERVINGS**

PREP TIME: 20 minutes
COOK TIME: 20 minutes
DRAINING TIME: 15 minutes

3 or 4 medium zucchini

Salt

1 or 2 garlic cloves, minced

¼ cup almond flour

2 eggs, whisked

Freshly ground black pepper

2 tablespoons butter

2 tablespoons sliced scallion, green parts only

PER SERVING: Calories: 101; Total carbs: 1g; **Net carbs: 1g, 5%; Total fat: 9g, 80%; Protein: 4g, 15%;** Fiber: 0g; Sugar: 0g

VARIATION 1: Calories: 115; Total carbs: 4g; **Net carbs: 2g, 14%; Total fat: 9g, 70%; Protein: 5g, 16%;** Fiber: 2g; Sugar: 2g

VARIATION 2: Calories: 101; Total carbs: 1g; **Net carbs: 1g, 5%; Total fat: 9g, 80%; Protein: 4g, 15%;** Fiber: 0g; Sugar: 0g

1. In a food processor or with a cheese grater, shred the zucchini into hash brown-like pieces. Transfer to a colander and sprinkle liberally with salt. Let sit in the sink for 15 to 20 minutes. Carefully rinse and drain the zucchini, pat dry with a paper towel, and place in a large bowl.

2. Add the garlic, almond flour, and eggs to the bowl. Season with pepper. Stir until well incorporated.

3. In a large skillet over medium-high heat, melt the butter. Spoon 2 to 3 tablespoons of the zucchini mixture into your hand and create a patty about half the size of your palm. Repeat with the remaining zucchini mixture. Carefully place the patties into the butter (you may have to cook these in batches). Cook for about 3 minutes until browned on one side. Flip and cook the other side for about 3 minutes until browned. Serve topped with the sliced scallion.

VARIATION 1 **CAULIFLOWER FRITTERS:** Boil the florets from 1 head cauliflower for 5 to 6 minutes. Drain and transfer to a food processor. Follow the rest of the recipe as written.

VARIATION 2 **BAKED ZUCCHINI FRITTERS:** Instead of panfrying these, make a big batch all at once and arrange them on a buttered baking sheet. Bake at 375°F for about 20 minutes, turning halfway through the cooking time, until browned.

PERFECT PAIR: Serve with Bacon Ranch Dip (page 24).

ZUCCHINI CHIPS

Making chips out of vegetables might be one of the easiest ways to get kids to eat their veggies—they're delicious and they're great for dipping. I started making veggie chips regularly when I got a mandoline—it made slicing so easy! I highly suggest getting this handy tool if you don't already have one; if not, slice carefully with a sharp knife. **MAKES 2 SERVINGS**

PREP TIME: 10 minutes
COOK TIME: 20 minutes

2 tablespoons olive oil

2 large zucchini, very thinly sliced

1 teaspoon onion powder

1 teaspoon garlic powder

Salt

Freshly ground black pepper

PER SERVING: Calories: 131; Total carbs: 2g; **Net carbs: 2g, 6%; Total fat: 14g, 92%; Protein: 1g, 2%;** Fiber: 0g; Sugar: 1g

VARIATION 1: Calories: 187; Total carbs: 3g; **Net carbs: 2g, 7%; Total fat: 18g, 84%; Protein: 5g, 9%;** Fiber: 1g; Sugar: 1g

VARIATION 2: Calories: 131; Total carbs: 2g; **Net carbs: 2g, 6%; Total fat: 14g, 92%; Protein: 1g, 2%;** Fiber: 0g; Sugar: 1g

1. In a large skillet over medium-high heat, heat the olive oil.

2. Working in batches, fry the zucchini chips for 3 to 4 minutes per side or until browned and beginning to crisp. Transfer to a paper towel–lined plate and sprinkle immediately with onion powder, garlic powder, salt, and pepper.

3. Repeat with the remaining zucchini slices and seasonings.

VARIATION 1 **BREADED ZUCCHINI CHIPS:** In a small bowl, whisk 1 egg. Dip the zucchini chips first in the egg and then into some almond flour before frying.

VARIATION 2 **OVEN-BAKED ZUCCHINI CHIPS:** Place the zucchini chips on a rimmed baking sheet. Drizzle with olive oil and season with salt, pepper, onion powder, and garlic powder. Bake at 375°F for 15 to 20 minutes, or until golden brown and crisp around the edges.

PERFECT PAIR: Serve with Low-Carb Ketchup (page 226) or Ranch Dressing (page 225) for dipping.

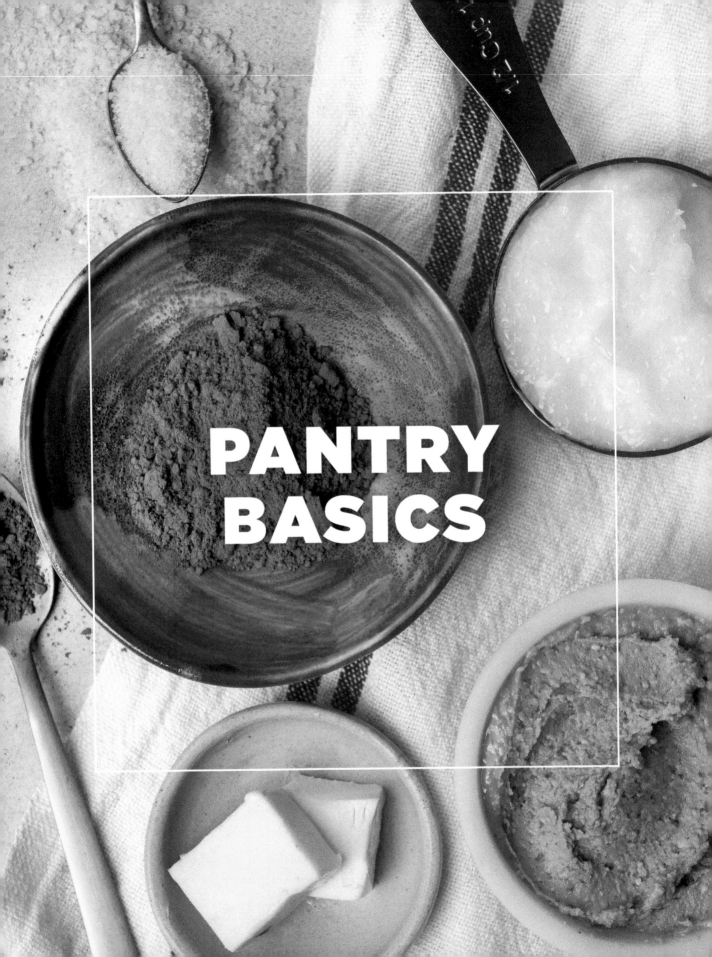

PANTRY BASICS

A ketogenic *pantry* is kind of an oxymoron—most staples you need for a keto diet are found in the refrigerator (eggs, meat, dairy, veggies), and the following recipes are no exception. Make these staples ahead and keep them on hand for snacks, sauces, and even drink options.

Having good keto snack options is the key to success. In my opinion, meals are easy enough; it's when you get hungry between breakfast and lunch or lunch and dinner that things can get tricky. Hopefully, this chapter gives you ideas to keep those between-meals cravings at bay.

BONE BROTH

I've always loved having bone broth ready to go, but it wasn't until I went keto that I really started enjoying it on a daily basis. Once used only as the broth in my soups, I soon found myself having a mug full of broth every morning, especially if I was doing intermittent fasting. I like to make a big batch, put some in the refrigerator, and freeze the rest in big cocktail ice-cube trays so I can just throw a couple in a mug and defrost them as needed. **MAKES 8 TO 10 SERVINGS**

PREP TIME: 10 minutes **COOK TIME:** 8 hours

1 pound bones from a roasted chicken, or beef bones

2 carrots, chopped

1 onion, quartered

2 garlic cloves, smashed

1. In a Dutch oven over high heat, combine the bones, carrots, onion, garlic, and enough water to cover the bones by 2 or 3 inches. Bring to a boil. Reduce the heat to low, cover the Dutch oven, and simmer for as long as possible, but at least 8 hours.

2. Pour the broth through a fine-mesh sieve to drain. Discard the bones and soggy vegetables. Refrigerate the broth if you plan to drink it within 1 week, otherwise freeze it in ice-cube trays and transfer to a freezer bag or container.

PER SERVING (1 cup): Calories: 37; Total carbs: 2g;
Net carbs: 2g, 22%; Total fat: 1g, 24%; Protein: 5g, 54%;
Fiber: 0g; Sugar: 0g

COCONUT BUTTER COFFEE

I make this coffee for myself most mornings, especially when I'm trying to be as strictly keto as possible. It's an amazing way to get your daily caffeine boost and also start the day with a large serving of fat, which usually keeps me full well into lunchtime. **MAKES 1 SERVING**

PREP TIME: 10 minutes **COOK TIME:** 5 minutes

1 cup hot coffee

1½ teaspoons unsalted butter

1 tablespoon coconut oil

1 teaspoon ground cinnamon (optional)

Prepare your coffee in your usual manner. Add the butter and coconut oil. Use a handheld frother or a blender to whip it until frothy. Sprinkle with the cinnamon (if using) and drink immediately.

PER SERVING: Calories: 170; Total carbs: 0g;
Net carbs: 0g, 0%; Total fat: 19g, 100%; Protein: 0g, 0%;
Fiber: 0g; Sugar: 0g

RANCH DRESSING

We go through quite a bit of ranch dressing in our house; I love dipping veggies into it or serving on the side with certain chicken dishes and on greens for a quick salad. It's really easy to make at home, which helps you cut down on the amount of preservatives you feed your family. If you want, make a big batch of the spice mix so it's ready to go when you need it (it's also a great way to season meat before grilling). **MAKES ABOUT 1½ CUPS**

PREP TIME: 5 minutes **COOK TIME:** 5 minutes

1 cup Keto Mayonnaise (to the right)

½ cup sour cream

1½ teaspoons dried chives

1 teaspoon dry mustard

½ teaspoon dried dill

½ teaspoon celery seed

½ teaspoon onion powder

½ teaspoon garlic powder

Salt

Freshly ground black pepper

In an airtight container with a lid, combine the mayonnaise, sour cream, chives, mustard, dill, celery seed, onion powder, and garlic powder. Season with salt and pepper. Stir well to combine and refrigerate until ready to use. This will keep for about 1 week.

PER SERVING (2 tablespoons): Calories: 43; Total carbs: 3g; **Net carbs: 2g, 28%; Total fat: 3g, 63%; Protein: 1g, 9%;** Fiber: 1g; Sugar: 2g

KETO MAYONNAISE

Mayonnaise is super keto-friendly. I make it myself to cut down on my soy consumption and all the preservatives that come in store-bought sauces such as mayo and ranch dressing. Mayo is terrific to keep on hand because you can use it to easily make delicious sauces like aioli. It's relatively easy to whip up, so I keep a jar in my refrigerator at all times.
MAKES ABOUT 1¼ CUPS

PREP TIME: 20 minutes **COOK TIME:** 10 minutes

1 egg

2 tablespoons freshly squeezed lemon juice

1 teaspoon dry mustard

½ teaspoon salt

1¼ cups light olive oil, divided
(use avocado oil if you prefer)

1. Let the egg and lemon juice come to room temperature for at least 20 minutes, and up to 2 hours, before using.

2. In a food processor, combine the egg, lemon juice, mustard, salt, and ¼ cup of olive oil. Process quickly to combine.

3. With the food processor running, slowly drizzle in the remaining 1 cup of olive oil. When you have about 2 tablespoons left, pour it in quickly.

4. Keep the mayonnaise refrigerated until the expiration date on the eggs you use (make a note on the container).

PER SERVING (2 tablespoons): Calories: 220; Total carbs: 0g; **Net carbs: 0g, 0%; Total fat: 24g, 98%; Protein: 1g, 2%;** Fiber: 0g; Sugar: 0g

HOLLANDAISE SAUCE

Most of the time, I make hollandaise sauce only if I'm making eggs Benedict (or Baked Eggs Florentine, page 18), but the super-rich, super-buttery sauce is great on all kinds of things, especially vegetables! Try dipping steamed broccoli or asparagus in it. This is one of the few recipes in this chapter that you have to make when you need it because it has to be kept warm until served, so don't try to make it ahead of time.

MAKES 4 SERVINGS

PREP TIME: 5 minutes **COOK TIME:** 10 minutes

4 egg yolks

1 tablespoon freshly squeezed lemon juice

½ cup (1 stick), unsalted butter, melted

¼ teaspoon ground cayenne pepper

Pinch salt

1. In a large heatproof bowl, whisk together the egg yolks and lemon juice until the mixture becomes frothy and starts to expand.

2. Place the bowl over a saucepan of simmering water (do not let the water touch the bowl) and continue to whisk.

3. While whisking, slowly drizzle in the melted butter and continue to whisk until the sauce doubles in size, 8 to 10 minutes.

4. Remove from the heat and add the cayenne and the salt. Serve immediately or keep warm until ready to serve.

PER SERVING (3 tablespoons): Calories: 259; Total carbs: 1g; **Net carbs: 1g, 1%; Total fat: 27g, 94%; Protein: 3g, 5%;** Fiber: 0g; Sugar: 0g

LOW-CARB KETCHUP

Ketchup is one of those sauces I never cared about until I went keto, and then, suddenly, I missed it. This Paleo ketchup is made without sugar, and it's really easy: you basically just season tomato paste with spices, add some vinegar and water, then let it chill in the refrigerator while the flavors blend together. Tomatoes are pretty high in carbs overall so, while this is a much better choice than store-bought ketchup, I recommend using it in moderation, especially if you're actively trying to lose weight.

MAKES ABOUT 6 SERVINGS

PREP TIME: 5 minutes
COOK TIME: 0 minutes
CHILLING TIME: 8 hours

1 (6-ounce) can tomato paste

⅓ cup water

2 tablespoons white vinegar

¼ teaspoon dry mustard

¼ teaspoon ground allspice

¼ teaspoon ground cinnamon

⅛ teaspoon ground cayenne pepper

1 tablespoon Swerve, or other low-carb sweetener

2 pinches salt

In a large jar, combine the tomato paste, water, vinegar, mustard, allspice, cinnamon, cayenne, Swerve, and salt. Stir well to combine. Cover and refrigerate for at least 8 hours before serving.

PER SERVING (2 tablespoons): Calories: 28; Total carbs: 6g; **Net carbs: 5g, 86%; Total fat: 0g, 0%; Protein: 1g, 14%;** Fiber: 1g; Sugar: 4g

ALMOND BUTTER "SNACK PACK"

This is my usual keto bedtime snack. It's really easy to make ahead of time so you can pack it for work or send your kids to school with it—with just a few ingredients, it's incredibly filling and so delicious. **MAKES 1 SERVING**

PREP TIME: 5 minutes

2 tablespoons almond butter

1 tablespoon coconut oil

5 fresh raspberries

1 tablespoon shredded coconut

In a small bowl, mix together the almond butter and coconut oil until smooth. Top with the raspberries and shredded coconut. Keep refrigerated in an airtight container for up to 1 week (though it's best when freshly made).

PER SERVING: Calories: 386; Total carbs: 16g; **Net carbs: 8g, 17%; Total fat: 34g, 79%; Protein: 8g, 4%;** Fiber: 10g; Sugar: 6g

COCONUT LEMON WATER

Sometimes, at the end of the day, I look at my macros and realize I'm a little short on fat, but I don't have enough protein/carbs/calories left for a snack, or I'm just not hungry enough to eat again. In these situations I turn to this coconut lemon water, which sounds a lot fancier than it really is. I find the acidity from the lemon makes the water feel a little less "oily," and I really enjoy it. **MAKES 1 SERVING**

PREP TIME: 5 minutes
COOK TIME: 5 minutes

8 to 10 ounces hot water

1 tablespoon coconut oil

1 lemon slice

Pour the water into a mug and add the coconut oil. Stir until melted. Add the lemon slice. Enjoy immediately.

PER SERVING: Calories: 117; Total carbs: 0g; **Net carbs: 0g, 0%; Total fat: 14g, 100%; Protein: 0g, 0%;** Fiber: 0g; Sugar: 0g

BASIC SWEET FAT BOMBS

This easy recipe is my go-to for sweet fat bombs. They contain just 5 core ingredients that you're likely to always have on hand. If you like them on the sweeter side, add a few drops of liquid stevia. **MAKES 5 LARGE FAT BOMBS OR 10 SMALL BOMBS**

PREP TIME: 5 minutes
COOK TIME: 30 minutes
CHILLING TIME: 15 to 20 minutes

½ cup coconut oil

½ cup unsweetened peanut butter

¼ cup unsweetened cocoa powder

1 to 2 tablespoons butter

2 or 3 drops liquid stevia (optional)

Pinch salt

1. In a small saucepan over low heat, melt the coconut oil. Add the peanut butter and stir well to combine. Stir in the cocoa powder and butter until smooth.

2. Remove the saucepan from the heat and pour the mixture into baking molds, such as silicone ice-cube trays or silicone cupcake liners, or use paper cupcake liners and peel them off.

3. Freeze the fat bombs for 15 to 20 minutes if you want to enjoy them soon, or refrigerate for 3 hours to cool and harden. Keep refrigerated in an airtight container for up to 2 weeks.

PER SERVING (½ large bomb or 1 small bomb): Calories: 203; Total carbs: 4g; **Net carbs: 2g, 8%; Total fat: 19g, 84%; Protein: 4g, 8%;** Fiber: 2g; Sugar: 1g

BASIC SAVORY FAT BOMBS

These savory fat bombs are basically just cream cheese bites, but you can do a lot with them if you switch up the coating. I love them with crumbled bacon or shredded Cheddar cheese (or a mixture of both), or crushed nuts or seeds (they're actually delicious dipped in the everything bagel seasoning from my Everything Bagel Cream Cheese Dip, page 55). **MAKES 8 FAT BOMBS**

PREP TIME: 10 minutes

8 ounces cream cheese, cold

Your choice of coatings: crumbled cooked bacon, shredded cheese, crushed pecans, etc.

Divide the cream cheese into 8 portions. Working quickly so as not to soften it too much, roll the cream cheese into small balls. Dip the balls in your preferred toppings and transfer back to the refrigerator for about 10 minutes, or until ready to serve. Keep refrigerated in an airtight container up until the expiration date on your cream cheese package (make a note on the container).

PER SERVING (1 bomb [base]): Calories: 102; Total carbs: 1g; **Net carbs: 1g, 4%; Total fat: 10g, 88%; Protein: 2g, 8%;** Fiber: 0g; Sugar: 0g

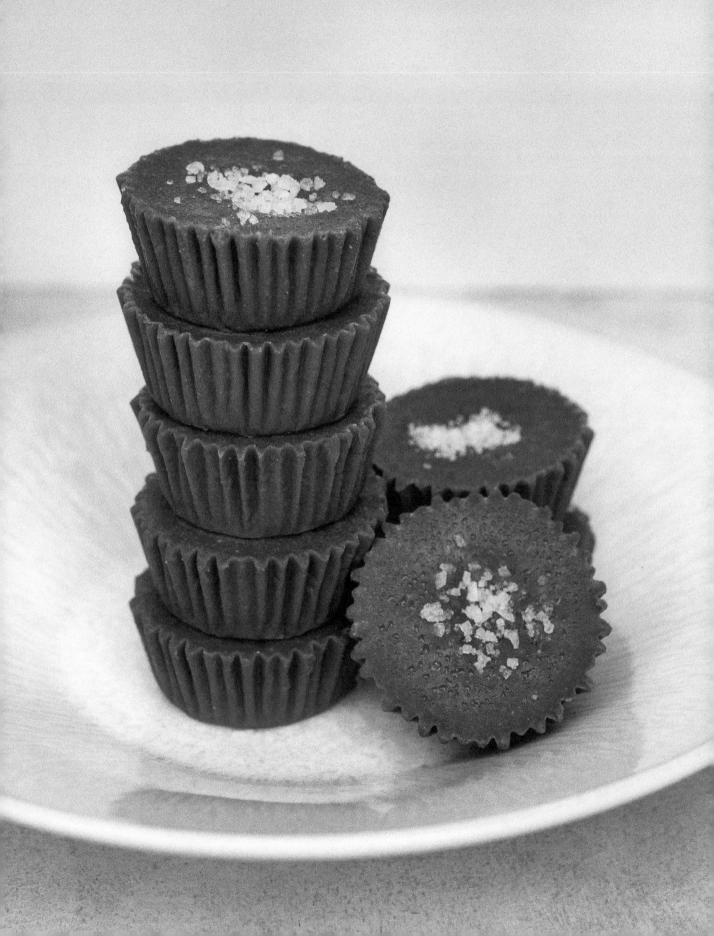

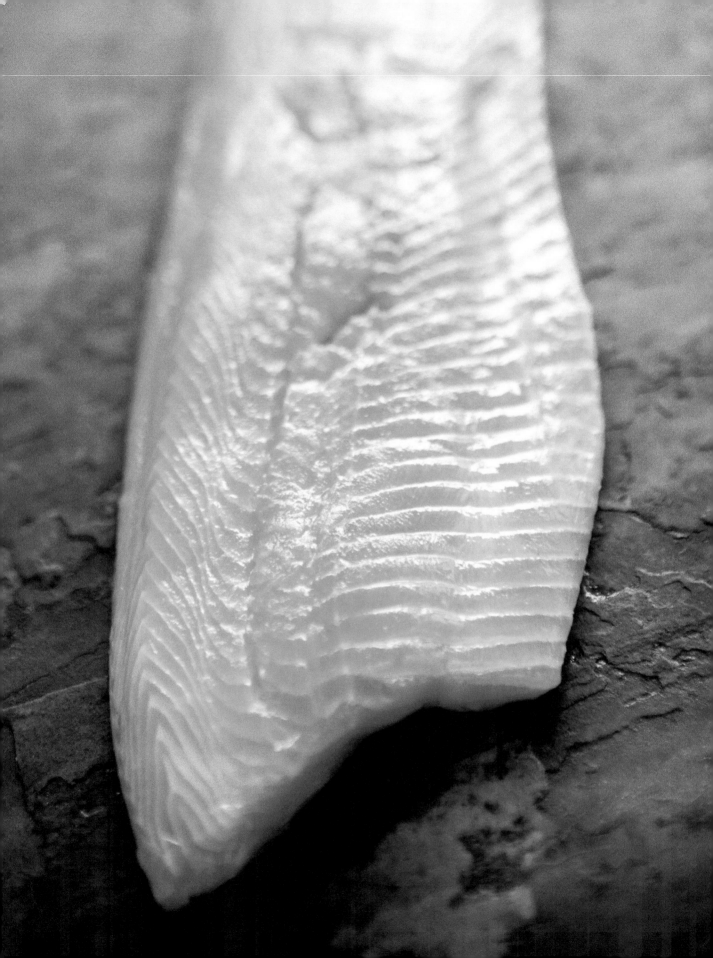

Measurement and Conversion Tables

VOLUME EQUIVALENTS (LIQUID)

STANDARD	US STANDARD (OUNCES)	METRIC (APPROXIMATE)
2 tablespoons	1 fl. oz.	30 mL
¼ cup	2 fl. oz.	60 mL
½ cup	4 fl. oz.	120 mL
1 cup	8 fl. oz.	240 mL
1½ cups	12 fl. oz.	355 mL
2 cups or 1 pint	16 fl. oz.	475 mL
4 cups or 1 quart	32 fl. oz.	1 L
1 gallon	128 fl. oz.	4 L

OVEN TEMPERATURES

FAHRENHEIT (F)	CELSIUS (C) (APPROXIMATE)
250°	120°
300°	150°
325°	165°
350°	180°
375°	190°
400°	200°
425°	220°
450°	230°

VOLUME EQUIVALENTS (DRY)

STANDARD	METRIC (APPROXIMATE)
⅛ teaspoon	0.5 mL
¼ teaspoon	1 mL
½ teaspoon	2 mL
¾ teaspoon	4 mL
1 teaspoon	5 mL
1 tablespoon	15 mL
¼ cup	59 mL
⅓ cup	79 mL
½ cup	118 mL
⅔ cup	156 mL
¾ cup	177 mL
1 cup	235 mL
2 cups or 1 pint	475 mL
3 cups	700 mL
4 cups or 1 quart	1 L

WEIGHT EQUIVALENTS

STANDARD	METRIC (APPROXIMATE)
½ ounce	15 g
1 ounce	30 g
2 ounces	60 g
4 ounces	115 g
8 ounces	225 g
12 ounces	340 g
16 ounces or 1 pound	455 g

Keto Diet Resources

- **Reddit.com/r/keto**
  A great forum for asking questions and reading about other people's experiences with keto. There's also a page for women on keto and even keto and pregnancy/fertility.

- **Ruled.me/keto-calculator**
  A keto calculator such as this one will help you plan out how much you should be eating and how much of it should be carbs, fat, and protein. This is the first step in starting this diet.

- **MyFitnessPal**
  This app is crucial to tracking your food and seeing what your macros look like every day. I used it religiously for a month or two and it really helped me learn the nutritional value of many of the foods I eat every day.

Recipe Index by Meal

Recipe Index

Index

About the Author

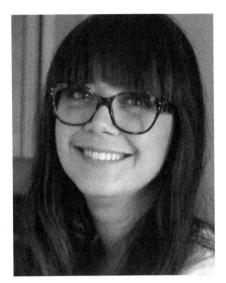

Megan Flynn Peterson is the writer behind *Freckled Italian*, a blog that focuses on life, love, and lots of food. She has called Virginia, Minnesota, and North Carolina home, but currently resides in the San Francisco Bay Area with her husband and their rescue pup as they await the arrival of their first child, a daughter due in late November 2017. This is her third cookbook. You can read more from Megan at FreckledItalian.com/blog, or find her on Instagram and Twitter @MFlynnPete.